T0144684

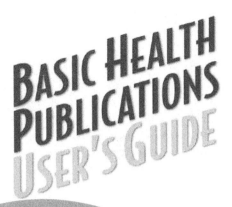

BASIC HEALTH
PUBLICATIONS
USER'S GUIDE

TO
CHROMIUM

*Don't Be a Dummy.
Become an Expert
on What Chromium
Can Do for Your
Health.*

MELISSA DIANE SMITH
JACK CHALLEM Series Editor

The information contained in this book is based upon the research and personal and professional experiences of the author. It is not intended as a substitute for consulting with your physician or other health care provider. Any attempt to diagnose and treat an illness should be done under the direction of a health care professional.

The publisher does not advocate the use of any particular health care protocol but believes the information in this book should be available to the public. The publisher and author are not responsible for any adverse effects or consequences resulting from the use of the suggestions, preparations, or procedures discussed in this book. Should the reader have any questions concerning the appropriateness of any procedures or preparation men-tioned, the author and the publisher strongly suggest consulting a professional health care advisor.

Series Editor: Jack Challem
Editor: Carol Rosenberg
Typesetter: Gary A. Rosenberg
Series Cover Designer: Mike Stromberg

Basic Health Publications User's Guides are published by Basic Health Publications, Inc.

CONTENTS

Introduction, 1

1. Basics about Chromium, 3

2. Nutritional Therapy for Diabetes, 10

3. A Protector against Cholesterol Problems, Syndrome X, and Heart Disease, 17

4. An Aid in Fighting the Battle of the Bulge, 23

5. An Antiaging Agent, 27

6. A Natural Remedy for Depression and Premenstrual Syndrome, 35

7. Other Benefits and Areas for Future Research, 46

8. How to Buy and Use Chromium, 57

9. Nutrients and Other Factors That Enhance Chromium's Effects, 68

Conclusion, 80

Selected References, 82

Other Books and Resources, 85

Index, 88

INTRODUCTION

Can a trace mineral make a huge difference in health? Absolutely, especially when that mineral is chromium. Needed in minute amounts by the body, chromium promotes optimal health by protecting against the most common chronic diseases in our modern world.

Why is chromium so health promoting? Chromium helps the blood–sugar-lowering hormone, insulin, function more efficiently. This benefit may seem minor or only important for diabetics, but it's important for all of us. Insulin, the master hormone of our metabolism, regulates the body's breakdown of carbohydrates, protein, and fats for energy. Obviously, the better insulin functions, the better the body functions.

We now know that most health problems and chronic diseases that plague the Western world are brought on by uncontrolled blood sugar and disturbances of insulin function. By helping insulin work more effectively, chromium combats these problems—not only several different types of diabetes, but also obesity, prediabetes, hypoglycemia, unhealthy cholesterol levels, high blood pressure, Syndrome X, and heart disease. By keeping insulin and blood sugar levels in check, chromium can also delay the effects of aging. It is even helpful in some cases of depression, premenstrual syndrome, seasonal affective disorder, and osteoporosis. In other words, chromium is a tiny nutrient that packs a mighty therapeutic punch for its size.

Nutritionally speaking, it's usually best to get nutrients from food whenever possible. However, chromium levels have been depleted from our soil, and few foods today have high amounts of chromium. Amazingly, 90 percent of Americans don't receive adequate amounts of chromium from their diets. What's more, most Americans eat excessive amounts of sugar and refined grains, which deplete chromium levels.

With most people running on low levels of chromium, it shouldn't be surprising that the incidences of insulin-related health conditions such as type II diabetes and obesity are at all-time highs. But they don't have to be. Insulin-related health problems are nutritional diseases that can be corrected and prevented with nutrition. One of the first places to start is with chromium supplementation.

All nutrients are important, but chromium may be a little extra important in this day and age. Delve into this book and find out the many reasons why.

CHAPTER 1

BASICS ABOUT CHROMIUM

Chromium is an essential nutrient that's needed for optimal blood sugar function. Lack of dietary chromium is widespread in industrialized nations and is a contributing factor in the development of many common blood–sugar- and insulin-related health problems.

A Mineral Needed in Small but Regular Amounts

Chromium is a mineral, not a vitamin. Vitamins and minerals are both necessary for health, but minerals are simpler in chemical form and are tiny in comparison to vitamins.

Unlike calcium and magnesium, which are found in large amounts in the body, chromium is a trace mineral found in minute amounts. It doesn't take much chromium to fulfill our basic need for this mineral. However, if we don't get the small amount we need, our health suffers.

Minerals
Elements that cannot be broken down into simpler substances. A trace mineral is one that is needed in very tiny amounts.

Chemistry: Nutritional versus Industrial Chromium

It should be pointed out that chromium in this book refers to nutritional chromium, which is technically known as trivalent chromium because it has a net electronic charge of plus three (+3). There is another type of chromium, hexavalent chromium (Cr6+), which I'll call industrial chromium, just to keep it simple. Industrial chromium forms as a byproduct of certain industrial processes, such as the making of stainless and hard-alloy steel.

If you saw the movie *Erin Brokovich*, you may recall that industrial or hexavalent chromium has been shown to cause cancer. But don't be alarmed: industrial chromium has nothing to do with nutritional chromium—and nutritional chromium cannot change into industrial chromium inside the body. There are numerous examples of substances having vastly different properties in different forms. For example, oxygen is health promoting in some forms, while it is hazardous to health in other forms.

Trivalent Chromium
The scientific name for nutritional chromium, the type of chromium we need for health.

If you read about chromium in scientific terms, here's how to keep the two forms straight: When you hear about hexavalent chromium, think of "hex" as something that brings you very bad luck. However, when you hear the prefix "tri" in trivalent chromium, think "Three's a charm." As you read this book, you'll learn just what kind of magic nutritional chromium can do for people with many different kinds of blood–sugar- and insulin-related health problems.

Chromium's Essentiality Discovered in the 1970s

By the 1950s, chromium was known to help control blood sugar in animals, but it wasn't until 1977 that chromium was proven to be essential for human health. Hospitalized patients who could not take in food by mouth were given Total Parental Nutrition (TPN)—a solution of all the nutrients they needed to maintain health—directly into their veins. Some of these patients developed high blood sugar levels and other diabetic-type symptoms. Doctors tried to start insulin therapy to treat the condition, but it didn't work very well.

Physicians got the idea that the patients were showing signs of chromium deficiency. Small amounts of chromium were added to the patients' intravenous feeding solutions. With the addition of this one nutrient, the patients quickly improved: their blood sugars and other abnormalities returned to normal. The Food and Drug Administration (FDA) and the Food and Nutrition Board of the National Research Council, therefore, designated chromium an essential trace mineral for human health.

The Relationship between Chromium and Insulin

To understand what happens when we don't get enough chromium, it's important to understand more about chromium and the hormone insulin.

Insulin is the master hormone of our metabolism. It controls blood sugar levels, regulates many aspects of the breakdown and utilization of carbohydrates, fats, and protein for energy, and directly affects certain genetic processes. Keeping insulin working correctly is an important factor in health.

Here's where chromium comes in: the trace mineral helps insulin work more efficiently to allow blood sugar (or glucose) to move from the blood into the cells. Glucose is a fuel that cells need for energy.

Researchers still don't know exactly how chromium does its magic, but it may help insulin at-

Insulin
A key metabolic hormone that lowers blood sugar levels by increasing the rate at which glucose is taken up by cells throughout the body.

tach more easily to the necessary molecular docks. Also, it may be involved in enzyme reactions that lead to increased insulin sensitivity (or receptivity). Regardless of the mechanism, without chromium, the blood–sugar-lowering hormone insulin won't work properly and blood sugar, in turn, will rise to unhealthy levels.

Insulin Resistance—The Root of Many Health Problems

Before blood sugar levels rise to consistently unhealthy levels, a condition called insulin resistance usually develops. Insulin resistance sneaks up on people over years and sometimes decades, primarily from eating the wrong foods and not getting enough nutrients.

Insulin Resistance
A condition in which the body does not respond to insulin efficiently. High insulin levels usually accompany insulin resistance.

What happens is this: Sugary treats and a lot of white-flour products provoke a steep rise in blood sugar. The body responds by releasing insulin to lower blood sugar to healthy levels. This works fine for a while; however, the more often blood–sugar-rising foods are eaten, the more the body has to pump out extra levels of insulin to keep blood sugar in a normal range.

Eventually, the body becomes overwhelmed by so much insulin that it doesn't respond as efficiently to insulin's blood–sugar-lowering effects. (This condition—insulin resistance—is very much like taking so much of a drug that it loses its effectiveness and a person needs a larger amount of it to get the same effect.) When insulin isn't working efficiently, the body compensates by churning out even greater insulin levels to keep glucose levels in check.

Chromium Fights High Insulin and High Blood Sugar

The combination of insulin resistance and high insulin levels can go on silently for years or decades without a person knowing it. Unfortunately, all the while, the excess insulin does damage and sets disease into motion inside the body. If this continues, blood sugar levels gradually rise, either because body cells become even less responsive to the action of insulin or because the workhorse pancreas eventually tires and stops producing adequate amounts of insulin.

Later in this book, you'll learn that both high insulin levels and high blood sugar levels are hazardous to health and contribute to premature aging. Fortunately, chromium protects against both conditions because it helps insulin work more effectively.

Chromium Needs Vary

The amount of chromium that people need varies. It depends primarily on their intake and state of health. Those who are most lacking in the nutrient need it the most.

The symptoms of chromium deficiency include elevated blood sugar, insulin, and cholesterol; elevated blood triglycerides; and decreased levels of the good HDL cholesterol. All of these conditions have been shown to respond well to chromium supplementation.

The Recommended Daily Allowance Committee recommends 50–200 mcg of chromium per day. This amount seems reasonable for the average healthy person, but higher amounts are needed for people with many conditions involving insulin resistance, such as type II diabetes and prediabetes.

50–200 mcg
The estimated safe and recommended amount of chromium the average healthy person needs on a daily basis.

Low Intakes Are Exceedingly Common

Unfortunately, most Americans don't obtain the minimum 50 mcg of chromium from their daily diets. Research from the USDA found that men average 33 mcg of chromium per day in their diets and women average 25 mcg per day—and the situation is similar in other countries. Even diets designed to be well balanced by nutritionists almost always contain less than 50 mcg of chromium.

What makes it so difficult to meet our needs for chromium? To begin with, only a few foods are rich sources of chromium. Second, our soil has been depleted of many minerals, including chromium; foods that grow in the depleted soil are therefore low in chromium and other minerals that we need.

The best sources of chromium are organ meats, oysters, broccoli, mushrooms, brewers yeast, brown rice, barley, and wheat germ. Unfortunately, the first two foods aren't widely eaten. Also, there are a large number of people who are susceptible to yeast infections or who have yeast or grain sensitivities and should therefore avoid or limit some of the other foods.

Our bodies are designed to thrive on an ample supply of chromium along with few or no foods that act as chromium depletors. Our Stone-Age ancestors regularly ate organ meats, so they likely had a higher intake of chromium than we have today. In addition, Stone-Age people ate no refined sugar or refined grains, which are very low in chromium and also promote chromium losses in the urine.

Chromium excretion also increases with infection, strenuous exercise, pregnancy, and stress, and we lose chromium as we age. The highest tissue levels of chromium are found in newborns; tissue levels decrease from then on throughout the rest of our lives. Because of all these factors—inadequate chromium intake, increased chromium losses, and decreasing chromium tissue levels as we age—virtually all of us can benefit from rebuilding the body's stockpile of chromium by taking chromium supplements.

In the chapters that follow, you'll read over and over again how chromium's ability to improve faulty insulin function carries considerable therapeutic weight against a wide variety of blood–sugar- and insulin-related conditions. We'll start the discussion by covering chromium's impressive health benefits for people with the most serious of these conditions, diabetes.

CHAPTER 2

NUTRITIONAL THERAPY FOR DIABETES

Diabetes can come in several different forms, but it's always characterized by abnormally high blood sugar levels. Diabetes is a serious disease that's out of sight and out of mind to many people, but it shouldn't be: it greatly increases the risk of coronary heart disease, stroke, blindness, nerve disorders, kidney disease, cancer, and impotence (in men). Moreover, the incidence of one particular type of diabetes, type II diabetes, is growing at an outstanding rate.

Improving insulin function to reduce blood sugar levels is the prime strategy for treating diabetes. Chromium improves insulin efficiency, so not surprisingly, chromium supplements have been found to be therapeutic for relieving symptoms and improving blood sugar and insulin levels in many different types of diabetes. Chromium also benefits the most common type of hypoglycemia (low blood sugar), which is often considered a precursor to type II diabetes.

The Different Types of Diabetes

Diabetes is generally classified into two main types, type I and type II. Type II is by far the most common type, accounting for 90 to 95 percent of all cases. Historically, this type of diabetes developed primarily in adults; therefore, it is often called adult-onset diabetes. Today, however, type II diabetes is developing in children at an alarming rate, including some children as young as ten years old. Primarily a disease brought on by an unhealthy diet and lifestyle, type II diabetes is insulin resistance in its worst form. Fortunately, it usually responds incredibly well to nutritional treatment.

Type I diabetes, also called insulin-dependent or juvenile-onset diabetes, is an autoimmune disease that usually develops in children or adults before age thirty. This type of diabetes isn't characterized by inefficient use of insulin but rather by a lack of insulin production. Something, perhaps a virus or a dietary factor, causes the immune system to destroy the insulin-producing cells in the pancreas.

Diabetes Mellitus

A condition caused by undersecretion of the hormone insulin (in type 1 diabetes) or cell insensitivity to insulin (in type II diabetes), leading to high blood glucose levels.

There also are a few types of diabetes that develop during stressful periods on the body. These include gestational diabetes (which develops during pregnancy) and drug-induced diabetes (which develops when people take certain drugs). The good news is that chromium has been found to be a helpful nutritional treatment for these many different types.

Chromium's Effectiveness in Type II Diabetes

Since chromium helps insulin to function better, researchers naturally suspected that supplemental chromium might help treat type II diabetes, the type in which insulin isn't used efficiently. Chromium, you'll recall, was deemed essential for human health after it was found to reverse diabetes in hospitalized patients. Research has found that chromium can do the same for large groups of type II diabetics.

Most of the studies involving supplemental

chromium for type II diabetes have shown positive results of one type or another. However, when one particular form of chromium—the most bioavailable form, chromium picolinate—has been used, *all* of the studies have yielded positive results (in blood sugar, blood insulin, and/or blood lipid [cholesterol and triglyceride] readings).

One of these studies, a 1997 study involving 180 type II diabetics in China, is a classic. It documented "spectacular" results in diabetics who took 500 mcg of chromium picolinate twice daily. After four months, nearly all of the diabetics no longer had traditional signs of diabetes. Their blood sugar and insulin levels dropped to near normal—something that medications could not achieve. Even more important, the "gold standard" diagnostic measure of diabetes—blood levels of hemoglobin A1c (sugar-damaged proteins that age cells)—also dropped to normal.

A follow-up study by some of the same researchers monitored 833 type II diabetics who took 500 mcg of chromium picolinate twice daily. A significant reduction in fasting blood sugar levels and in post-meal blood sugar levels was found during the ten months of the study. No negative side effects were shown from taking the supplements. In addition, more than 85 percent of the patients reported improvements in the common diabetic symptoms of excessive thirst, frequent urination, and fatigue.

Type II Diabetics Have Higher Needs for Chromium

It's important to understand that type II diabetics have altered chromium metabolism—greater excretion of chromium, lower tissue levels of chromium, and less of an ability to convert chromium to a usable form in the body. For all of these reasons, chromium supplements are a must for diabetics.

Supplements usually work very well if taken in high enough doses and effective forms. But the dose and form really makes a big difference. Type II diabetics who have taken chromium picolinate in low doses—200 mcg per day—have had some improvements in their condition; however, they have not had the same spectacular results as type II diabetics who have taken 1,000 mcg per day.

There's one big caveat about taking chromium supplements: *If you're a diabetic who takes insulin injections or sugar-lowering drugs, you should not take chromium supplements without working with a knowledgeable doctor who can help you safely adjust the dosages of your medications.* Supplemental chromium works so well at improving insulin function that less medication usually is needed. (And, sometimes, medication can be eliminated completely over time.) This is a good thing—it indicates a reversal or lessening of insulin resistance—but it also means that you should work with your doctor to carefully monitor your condition and avoid overmedicating yourself.

Chromium picolinate is very beneficial by itself for type II diabetics, but there appears to be a nutrient combination that's even more effective. That combination is chromium picolinate plus biotin, a B vitamin. Recent research indicates that this combination of nutrients stimulates greater blood sugar usage and greater improvements in cholesterol readings compared with those seen when chromium picolinate is taken alone. You'll learn more about this synergistic combination in Chapter 9.

Chromium Helps Prevent Type II Diabetes in Those at Risk

Although the incidence of type II diabetes is increasing in record numbers, many people don't yet have diabetes but are at high risk for developing it. Chromium supplements can help in these cases, too.

A study directed by William Cefalu, M.D., of Wake Forest University, monitored individuals at risk—people who were moderately obese and had a family history of diabetes. Some people received a placebo; others, 1,000 mcg of chromium picolinate daily. After four months of treatment with chromium, insulin resistance was reduced by 40 percent. Insulin resistance, you'll recall, is the condition at the core of type II diabetes. Chromium supplements, therefore, help reverse the underlying disease process that leads to type II diabetes. In other words, they help both prevent and reverse type II diabetes.

Chromium Helps Type I Diabetes, Too

Many diabetics who inject insulin—both type I diabetics and type II diabetics who are in more advanced stages of the disease—respond positively to chromium picolinate supplementation. About 70 percent of both types show improved insulin responsiveness after taking 200 mcg of supplemental chromium per day. Some experience such an improvement in insulin sensitivity that they are able to reduce the amount of insulin they inject or the amount of other blood–sugar-lowering medications they take.

Chromium can't cure type I diabetes—in other words, it can't make type I diabetics produce more insulin. But chromium helps make the injected insulin taken by type I diabetics work more effectively, so less is often needed. Therefore, type I diabetics, like type II diabetics, should monitor their condition carefully and work with their physicians regarding the appropriate dosages of their medications.

Chromium and Other Types of Diabetes

Chromium supplementation has been found to be helpful for still other types of diabetes. Gestational diabetes is a transitional diabetes that develops during pregnancy and can cause numerous health problems, including loss of the child. It's the most common medical complication of pregnancy today. Just eight weeks of supplementation with chromium picolinate can significantly improve glucose intolerance and reduce blood sugar and insulin levels in those with gestational diabetes, thereby reducing the risk of health problems for both the mother and her child.

The use of certain pharmaceutical drugs, such as corticosteroids or Thiazide diuretics, lead to significant chromium losses and can also sometimes induce diabetic-type conditions. Fortunately, chromium supplementation can lead to improvements in the body's handling of blood sugar in both cases. In one study, steroid-induced diabetes was ameliorated in thirty-eight of forty-one patients following supplementation with 200 mcg of chromium three times per day. This occurred even though blood–sugar-lowering drugs were reduced by 50 percent in all patients who were given chromium supplements.

A Blood Sugar Balancer That's Helpful for Hypoglycemia, Too

It is important to keep in mind that chromium is a nutrient, not a drug. Chromium helps insulin function more efficiently. It benefits people with all types of blood sugar and insulin disorders—not just people with insulin resistance and diabetes, but also people with reactive hypoglycemia (those who experience quick blood sugar highs followed by quick blood sugar lows). Reactive hypoglycemia may seem very different from diabetes, but it represents the beginning stages of blood sugar imbalance or glucose intolerance and is considered a precursor to diabetes.

Reactive Hypoglycemia
A condition character-ized by unstable blood sugar and symptoms such as mood and energy swings, sugar cravings, anxiety, and trembling.

In people with reactive hypoglycemia, supplemental chromium normalizes insulin function, leading to increased insulin efficiency and a return to normal glucose levels more quickly after a high-sugar in-take. It also alleviates hypo-glycemic symptoms, including sweating, trembling, blurred vision, and sleepiness. In people with diabetes, improved insulin efficiency leads to a more efficient removal of sugar from the blood and reduction of diabetic markers, such as hemoglobin A1c levels. It also leads to a reduction of diabetic symptoms, such as increased thirst, fre-quent urination, and fatigue. Chromium, therefore, can be considered a blood sugar balancer as well as a blood sugar regulator.

Chromium is not a magic bullet, however. Dia-betes and blood sugar problems can be due to many different factors. Chromium deficiency (even if it is just marginal) is one of those factors, but not the only one.

As you've learned, in many of the studies, chromium supplementation by itself is often quite effective in alleviating many different types of glu-cose intolerance. Sometimes, however, it is not. The best approach involves taking chromium supple-ments as well as taking supplements of other nutri-ents important for proper blood sugar and insulin function; eating a protein-rich, low-carbohydrate diet rich in vegetables; reducing stress; and being physically active. More information on these syner-gistic strategies will be covered in Chapter 9.

CHAPTER 3

A PROTECTOR AGAINST CHOLESTEROL PROBLEMS, SYNDROME X, AND HEART DISEASE

Insulin resistance and high insulin levels are major risk factors for heart disease. In addition, these conditions either directly or indirectly lead to other strong risk factors for heart disease, including upper-body ("apple-shaped" or abdominal) obesity; abnormal blood fat levels (that is, high triglycerides and high cholesterol or poor ratios of high-density lipoprotein to low-density lipoprotein cholesterol); and high blood pressure. This cluster of symptoms is known as Syndrome X.

Chromium helps improve insulin function so it's a critical nutrient for preventing and treating Syndrome X and thereby protecting against heart disease.

What Is Syndrome X?

Syndrome X
Insulin resistance plus abdominal obesity, high blood pressure, high blood triglycerides, and/or unhealthy blood cholesterol levels.

Syndrome X may sound mysterious but millions of Americans have Syndrome X and don't know it. The term refers to a group of conditions many Americans are very familiar with: abdominal obesity (a "spare tire" around the middle); high blood pressure; high blood triglycerides; and high blood cholesterol levels or poor HDL-to-LDL cholesterol ratios. These heart disease risk factors tend to occur together—that's why they're called a "syndrome." Sixty-five to 70 million Americans are estimated to have this syndrome.

Each of the components of Syndrome X increases the risk of heart disease and diabetes. A combination of two or more of these components has an additive, or cumulative, effect in increasing the risk all the more.

The Chromium Connection to Syndrome X

Insulin resistance is at the root of Syndrome X; hence, Syndrome X is sometimes called the insulin resistance syndrome. It should be thought of as a prediabetic condition.

Chromium helps insulin work properly and helps reverse insulin resistance. Therefore, it gets to the root of the problem and helps reverse Syndrome X, just as it does with type II diabetes.

The symptoms of chromium deficiency are actually the symptoms of Syndrome X—high blood sugar, high insulin, high cholesterol, high triglycerides, and low levels of the "good" HDL cholesterol. A lack of chromium can cause all these conditions, so it makes sense that supplemental chromium can help improve these conditions. You'll learn that chromium does indeed do this.

Chromium and Fat Metabolism

Chromium is important for fat metabolism as well as for carbohydrate metabolism. Numerous studies have found that chromium supplements have beneficial effects on blood fats—including decreasing high total cholesterol and high LDL cholesterol, increasing beneficial HDL cholesterol, and decreasing triglycerides.

One double-blind, placebo-controlled study found that dietary supplementation with chromium picolinate for two months lowered blood levels of triglycerides in diabetics by an average of 17.4 percent. Another study by Richard Anderson, M.D., and his colleagues at the USDA observed a 15-percent decrease in total cholesterol when type II diabetics were given 1,000 mcg of chromium picolinate per day. Since elevated triglycerides and elevated cholesterol are risk factors for heart disease, chromium's ability to favorably influence them makes the mineral important in the prevention of cardiovascular disease, especially for diabetics who are at increased risk.

Chromium Acts as a Cholesterol Normalizer

Not all studies have found that chromium supplements lower blood cholesterol. This is likely because of two reasons. One, it takes a while, sometimes several months, to improve insulin sensitivity and high blood cholesterol levels. Studies that have not found cholesterol-lowering effects from chromium supplementation have lasted fewer than six weeks.

Two, chromium seems to act as a cholesterol normalizer instead of an overall cholesterol reducer. Gilbert Kaats, Ph.D., of the Health and Medical Research Foundation in San Antonio, Texas, designed an innovative study to examine this effect. He grouped people according to their cholesterol levels; then he gave them 400 mcg of chromium picolinate daily. He found that people who already had high cholesterol levels (greater than 199 mg/dl) experienced a drop in blood cholesterol of 17 mg/dl. In people who had normal cholesterol levels (150–199 mg/dl), the levels didn't change. And in people with low cholesterol levels (less than 150 mg/dl), chromium supplementation raised blood cholesterol by 8 mg/dl.

Therefore, just as chromium acts as a normalizer of blood sugar levels (helping people with both diabetes and hypoglycemia), it also acts as a normalizer of cholesterol levels, reducing cholesterol levels if they are too high but increasing them if they are too low.

Most people are concerned about high blood cholesterol levels, but few know that there are dangers in having low blood cholesterol levels. Research has shown that cholesterol levels below 150 mg/dl are associated with an increased risk of stroke, depression, violence, and suicide. Therefore, it's beneficial to health to raise cholesterol if it is too low, reduce cholesterol if it is too high, and maintain cholesterol if it is in the normal range. That's exactly what chromium supplements do.

This chapter focuses on reversing Syndrome X and preventing heart disease, so lowering high cholesterol levels is the most applicable part. But it's reassuring to know that chromium doesn't lower cholesterol levels in everyone. It simply promotes healthy cholesterol levels. In addition, those who need chromium the most respond to supplemental chromium the best.

Chromium's Effect on Blood Pressure

For many decades, high blood pressure was called "essential hypertension," which meant that the cause was not known. However, research over the past few decades has changed all that, showing that most hypertension is caused by excessive insulin.

Insulin can increase blood pressure in numerous ways. The hormone can increase the retention of sodium, which can raise blood pressure. Insulin also excites the body's sympathetic nervous system, which in turn speeds up the heart rate and raises blood pressure. And it increases the secretion of the stress hormone cortisol, which constricts blood vessels and can promote high blood pressure.

Chromium's ability to augment insulin sensitivity,

therefore, can fix the root cause of many cases of high blood pressure. Animal studies at Georgetown University suggest that eating sugar raises blood pressure, but chromium picolinate supplements reduce typical sugar-induced elevations in blood pressure—at least up to a point. The best strategy for correcting hypertension, of course, is to take chromium supplements *and* to avoid eating sugar.

Chromium's Effect on Overweight

Chromium's role in helping overweight and obese people slim down will be covered in detail in the next chapter. Right now, let's cover a few basics.

The majority of Americans are now overweight and one-quarter are obese. Upper-body, "apple-shaped" obesity—seen often as a potbelly or beer belly—is a hallmark of Syndrome X, and it greatly increases the risk of heart disease and diabetes.

Upper Body Obesity

Extra weight carried through the middle of the body, often seen as a potbelly or beer belly. It's a common indicator of Syndrome X.

Insulin is a hormone that promotes the storage of fat when in excess. The higher insulin levels are, the more your body will pack on the pounds. Lowering insulin levels will help you burn fat and lose weight because you won't have the hormone working against you.

As already mentioned, most Americans don't get adequate chromium from their diets. They also eat excessive amounts of sugar and white-flour products, which deplete chromium levels in the body and raise blood sugar levels. Over time, the typical American diet leads to insulin resistance and high insulin levels, which in turn can lead to obesity.

It makes sense that the only way to break this vicious cycle is to start a program that improves insulin efficiency and lowers high insulin levels—first, by eating a lower-carbohydrate, protein-rich, vegetable-rich diet, and second, by taking chromium supplements.

Chromium—An Integral Part of an Anti-X Plan

Chromium doesn't act as a magic weight loss pill or a cholesterol- or blood–pressure-lowering drug (which is good because it doesn't come with any side effects!). Instead, it's a nutrient that combats all of the components of Syndrome X because it corrects the underlying problem—faulty insulin function.

Chromium supplements are indispensable for the nutritional treatment—and prevention—of Syndrome X. However, they're best used together with a blood–sugar-balancing diet and supplements of other nutrients important for proper blood sugar and insulin function (which you'll learn more about in Chapter 9).

As the coauthor of *Syndrome X: The Complete Nutritional Program to Prevent and Reverse Insulin Resistance* (John Wiley & Sons), I have put many clients on this type of nutrition plan and have also gotten feedback from many readers. The conclusion: An Anti-X™ nutrition plan, including chromium supplements, is very effective at improving heart-disease risk factors—or Syndrome X—all across the board.

When insulin resistance is reversed and numerous heart-disease risk factors fall by the wayside, the risk of developing heart disease and diabetes drops dramatically. Besides that, people who conquer Syndrome X feel more energetic and mentally focused—and look better—because insulin is functioning the way it should. The next chapter will cover the many ways chromium can help make it easier to lose weight and firm up the body.

CHAPTER 4

AN AID IN FIGHTING THE BATTLE OF THE BULGE

Sixty percent of Americans are now overweight, 25 percent are obese, and the numbers increase every year. Some experts believe that if something isn't done soon to correct this trend, nearly everyone will be overweight by the year 2020. Overweight and obesity greatly increase the risk of chronic diseases, such as type II diabetes, and are therefore public health problems.

For most people, going on a lower-carbohydrate diet is important for stimulating weight loss, but taking chromium supplements is another good bet for firming up and losing unwanted fat. Chromium can help fight the battle of the bulge on several fronts.

Better Functioning Insulin Means Better Fat Burning

Chromium's key role, again, is it helps insulin work efficiently. When insulin is working properly, the fat-burning mechanisms of the body operate optimally. Less insulin is needed to do its job, so the body produces less insulin. Important body processes—thermogenesis (the production of heat by the body through the burning of sugar or fat) and the basal metabolic rate (the rate at which the body spends energy for the maintenance activities of the body)—hum along efficiently, so there's little chance for energy to be stored as fat.

When insulin doesn't do its job properly, all of

this is reversed. More fat-promoting insulin is pumped out, the body's fat-burning processes are inhibited, and it's next to impossible to lose fat and get lean and trim. This is a common occurrence today because most people aren't getting adequate chromium and are eating foods that lead to further chromium losses.

Chromium Can Increase Lean Body Mass

When most people try to lose weight, they starve themselves on low-calorie diets, which cause a loss of lean body mass and a substantial decrease in their metabolic rates. Dieters following low-calorie diets, therefore, can lose weight, but they lose more muscle than fat and often become weak. Their metabolisms also slow down so they have a tendency to easily regain weight after they go off low-calorie diets.

The name of the game in weight control is not so much what you weigh as how much muscle you have compared with how much fat. (Lean muscle tissue actually weighs more than fat.)

Chromium, fortunately, can prevent loss of lean muscle tissue when a person moderately restricts calories. Better yet, when a person doesn't restrict calories, chromium can increase a person's total lean body mass. This in turn increases metabolism and the body's ability to burn fat.

Chromium helps maintain or build muscle mass because it's a potentiator of insulin. Among the many jobs insulin has, insulin directs amino acids (protein components) into muscle cells to build muscle. It also slows the breakdown or catabolism of body protein. When you're trying to lose weight, you want to lose fat but maintain or build muscle. Chromium supplements help you do that.

Exercise also increases insulin sensitivity, so physical activity and chromium supplementation often can work together to promote a trimmer, stronger body. Working out, however, increases a person's excretion of chromium, increasing his or her need for extra supplemental chromium.

Chromium Improves Body Composition

Several double-blind, placebo-controlled studies have shown that chromium supplementation stimulates fat loss, increases lean body mass, and helps lower body weight. In college-aged male weight lifters, male football players, and male and female swimmers, increases in lean body mass and reductions in body fat have been documented in those who have taken chromium supplements.

Chromium seems to be helpful for improving body composition in obese people, too. One 1998 study—after controlling for differences in calorie intake and expenditure among subjects—found that compared with those who received a placebo, obese subjects who received 400 mcg of chromium per day lost significantly more weight and fat, and had a greater loss in their percentage of body fat, without any loss of lean body mass. Supplemental chromium, therefore, can gradually improve body composition, but it often takes several months to see significant effects.

Even more exciting, a new combination of chromium picolinate and three other natural ingredients seems to magnify and quicken positive effects in weight and fat loss. You'll learn more about this new product in Chapter 9.

Chromium Reduces Sugar Cravings

By improving insulin sensitivity and keeping blood

sugar levels more even, chromium also reduces cravings for sugar and refined white-flour products. This is important because carbohydrate cravings and chromium deficiency tend to form a vicious cycle.

When the body has low levels of chromium, cravings for sugars and heavily refined grain products increase. People then give in to the cravings and eat those foods, but the more sweets they eat, the more they deplete chromium stores in the body. With even lower levels of chromium, cravings for more sweets develop and the unhealthy cycle can go on and on.

Fortunately, chromium can come to the rescue and stop this process. For example, some of my clients tell me they have had a lifelong sweet tooth, but when they start taking chromium supplements, their urges to eat sweets dramatically diminish. The more they stay away from sweets, the more they can build up their chromium reserves—and the more they do this, the easier it is for them to lose weight and look great.

In sum, chromium supplements aren't magic pills that automatically make people thinner and firm - er. However, they do a lot to help people lose fat and improve body composition, particularly in conjunction with a good diet (and moderate physical activity).

CHAPTER 5

An Antiaging Agent

Antiaging therapy is the rage these days, but most of the information written in this area is misleading. The truth is aging is inevitable: nothing can keep us young forever. But there's a lot we can do to age slowly and gracefully and delay or avoid developing the common chronic diseases of aging.

High insulin and high blood sugar levels—two factors that develop over time from eating the typical American diet—age us faster than anything else. Chromium brings down high insulin and high blood sugar and, therefore, plays a critical role in delaying the aging process.

Type II Diabetes—A Model of Accelerated Aging

To understand how chromium helps slow the aging process, it's important to know more about diabetes and the dangers of high insulin and high blood sugar.

Researchers see type II diabetes as a model of accelerated aging. Why is this? Because diabetics develop risk factors, symptoms, and chronic diseases of aging (such as heart disease) earlier in life than nondiabetics, and they generally die of chronic diseases at younger ages. Chromium supplements help prevent and reverse type II diabetes, a prime risk factor for heart disease and many other potentially fatal health consequences. So, for this simple reason alone, they hold back the aging process.

In addition, a decline in glucose tolerance is one of the changes normally associated with aging. Chromium supplementation is indispensable for improving glucose tolerance, so it holds back the aging process in this way, too.

The Aging Effects of High Insulin

We now know that the high insulin levels and high blood sugar levels that characterize type II diabetes both accelerate the aging process. You don't have to have diabetes to have either or both of these conditions and be on the fast track to aging. If you eat a diet that causes your body to pump out high levels of insulin—say, you're overweight around the middle—you're also aging prematurely.

Insulin is a powerful mitogen—it stimulates the division of cells and the activation of genes. Prolonged exposure to high levels of insulin, therefore, actually accelerates the aging of cells or makes cells act like older (instead of younger) cells. High insulin levels, it turns out, have their hand in the development of numerous age-related, chronic conditions— not just heart disease and type II diabetes, but also cognitive disorders, impaired thinking processes, dementia, Alzheimer's disease, and liver, pancreatic, endometrial, breast, and colorectal cancers.

The Aging Effects of
High Blood Sugar

High blood sugar (or high glucose) also does damage in the body. First, high blood sugar generates a lot of free radicals—destructive molecules that damage and age cells. The more free radicals there are in the body—without an equal balance of protective antioxidants, molecules that quench free radicals—the faster that cells are damaged and the body ages.

Second, high blood sugar reacts with and damages proteins in organs and tissues, forming "advanced glycation end-products." The abbreviation for these substances, AGEs, is appropriate: AGEs toughen proteins and quite literally age cells.

Blood sugar that combines with the protein hemoglobin in your blood is glycosylated hemoglobin or hemoglobin A1c. AGEs are also involved in clouding the proteins in the lens of the eye (forming cataracts), and in the development of wrinkled skin and

Hemoglobin A1c
Sugar-damaged hemoglobin. A marker that diabetics measure in their blood to monitor control of their condition.

stiff joints. Often it's the combination of lots of AGEs and lots of free radicals that leads to so many of the complications of type II diabetes.

With blood sugar, you don't just run into trouble if your fasting blood sugar levels are high enough to qualify as diabetes (above 125 mg/dl). Prediabetic blood sugar levels (above 110 but below 125) greatly increase the risk of heart disease and diabetes—two of the most common diseases of aging. In addition, fasting blood sugar levels in the upper range of normal (say, 109) substantially increase the risk of death from heart disease than in someone with blood sugar readings at the lower range of normal (say, 80). The more you can lower blood sugar readings toward optimal levels, the least likely you are to age prematurely.

Chromium Lowers High Insulin and High Blood Sugar

Through its ability to improve insulin efficiency, chromium lowers high blood sugar and insulin levels, staving off the consequences from these conditions that promote aging. Even if supplemental chromium reduces blood sugar and insulin levels just slightly, it reduces the risk of age-related disease a little. Therefore, taking chromium supplements can help delay aging.

Animal research bears this out: Rats deprived of chromium have shorter life spans, while rats supplemented with chromium picolinate live 37 percent longer than they do in their natural habitat.

The rats that live longer because of chromium supplementation have lower blood sugar, lower insulin, and lower blood levels of hemoglobin A1c—the marker that indicates good diabetic control and normal aging. Once again, supplemental chromium enhances insulin sensitivity, and by doing that, it helps maintain more youthful cell performance.

Supplemental Chromium— A Bit Like Caloric Restriction

The effect of supplemental chromium is very similar to that of caloric restriction on aging. To explain, researchers have known since the 1930s that restricting an animal's lifelong caloric intake by one-third extends its life span by one-third. Eating less protects against diabetes—and it also slows the aging process.

Currently, researchers at the University of Wisconsin, Madison, are applying caloric restriction to monkeys (not just rodents). Monkeys are biologically very similar to humans. While this experiment is still in progress, the researchers have reported that the calorie-restricted monkeys are showing no signs of type II diabetes and are acting, in effect, like young monkeys. In contrast, monkeys that are allowed to eat as much as they want—as many people do—are developing the early signs of diabetes.

Now, you're probably asking, what does caloric

restriction have to do with chromium? The answer is simple. If you would like to add a few years to your life, would you prefer to do it by cutting your calorie intake by one-third and always being a little hungry, or would you prefer to eat a normal calorie intake (that is, not overeat) and just take some chromium supplements?

Chromium can complement the beneficial effects of a lower-carbohydrate, lower-sugar diet to delay aging and likely add years to your life. Not only that, it will probably help you feel younger during those extra years.

Supplemental Chromium Raises DHEA Levels

Hormones have a powerful effect on body function, and chromium supplementation helps in a key way to keep our bodies hormonally younger: it helps increase the body's production of dehydroepiandrosterone (DHEA). One study found that after taking chromium supplements for a month, the DHEA levels of postmenopausal women increased to levels that would be typical of thirty- to thirty-five-year-old women.

This is significant because DHEA levels are perhaps the most telling of all the markers for aging. People with higher DHEA levels live longer and feel better: they have a greater sense of overall well-being and a better ability to deal with emotional and physical stress.

DHEA
A key hormone in the body that pro-motes youthful body function. Its production is suppressed when insulin levels are high.

On the other hand, the lower people's DHEA levels are, the more likely they are to develop degenerative diseases of accelerated aging, including hardening of the arteries, diabetes, cancer, osteoporosis, and lowered immunity. In addition, they're more likely to die from an age-related disease. For example, one 1986 *New England Journal of Medicine* study found that men with low DHEA levels were 3.3 times more likely to die of heart disease than those with normal levels.

Your body's levels of DHEA peak when you're in your twenties. After that, the amount of DHEA you produce declines at the rate of about 2 percent a year. By the time you're forty, you make only about half the DHEA you did at age twenty, and at age sixty-five, your level is only 10 to 20 percent of what it was at its peak.

Insulin, more than anything else, will suppress your natural DHEA production. Keeping insulin levels low—by following a lower-carbohydrate diet and taking chromium supplements—is one of the best ways to maintain a high DHEA level. If you do that, you keep the intricate network of hormones in your body functioning in a more youthful way.

The Hormone Connection to Aging

With the main exception of insulin (which can rise if we eat the wrong foods and don't take our chromium supplements), levels of virtually every other hormone in our bodies decline as we age. Hormones regulate every aspect of our bodies' functions, from metabolism to body temperature to sex drive. When levels of most hormones decline, youthful body function declines, too. When levels of those same hormones stay higher, the body functions as if it were younger.

Hormones
Powerful messenger chemicals that regulate body functions and are made by the endocrine glands, such as the pancreas, adrenals, and sex organs.

Made by the adrenal glands, DHEA is the precursor or source for other adrenal hormones, including the stress hormone cortisol, and all the sex hormones, such as estrogen, progesterone, and testosterone. It's often called the "mother" hormone for this very reason.

Clearly, if your body's production of DHEA declines, the cascade of hormone production that follows will be seriously disrupted, too. A steady drop in your hormone levels ushers in older body function and symptoms of aging, such as decreased resistance to infection, brittle bones, loss of muscle mass and tone, diminished libido, lower stamina, and trouble with short-term memory.

A drop in hormone production and a decline in mental and physical function are considered a natural part of aging, but you can do a lot to slow this process. If you maintain high DHEA levels—or raise DHEA levels if they're low—you automatically help your body improve its production of numerous hormones that keep it functioning more youthfully. You may feel decades younger and people may say you look and act decades younger than your chronological age.

Of course, many people today take DHEA supplements for this very reason, but DHEA supplements really shouldn't be taken without the supervision of a doctor. If too much DHEA is taken, it can throw off the whole intricate web of hormone function in the body, sometimes causing side effects, such as acne and excessive growth of facial hair in women. The far safer route to improve DHEA levels and feel better is to do it the natural way by taking chromium supplements, eating a lower-carbohydrate diet, and reducing stress.

Chromium Gets to the Roots of Aging

A lot of information has been covered in this chapter, but it boils down to this: an excess of free radicals and advanced glycation end-products, rising blood pressure, and diminishing levels of DHEA and other hormones all have been implicated in the aging process. Chromium positively influences all of these factors because it improves insulin sensitivity and lowers blood sugar and insulin levels.

Chromium supplementation extends the lifespan of rats, and all evidence suggests that it can do the same for us. Our modern lifestyle promotes high blood sugar and insulin levels, which are at the root of aging. Supplemental chromium can make a major dent in combating those roots. When combined with a lower-carbohydrate diet, some antioxidant supplements (which you'll learn more about in Chapter 9), physical activity, and stress reduction, taking chromium supplements is the closest thing we've found to a natural fountain of youth.

CHAPTER 6

A NATURAL REMEDY FOR DEPRESSION AND PREMENSTRUAL SYNDROME

Chromium normalizes blood sugar, and people with minor and major blood sugar disturbances often report increased mental focus and steadier moods from chromium supplementation. Recently, though, supplemental chromium has shown promising results in an exciting new area: the treatment of depression and premenstrual syndrome.

There are many different varieties and underlying causes of depression and premenstrual syndrome. Supplemental chromium isn't a panacea for all types of these conditions, but it has been found to be helpful for several types, both when used alone and when used with antidepressant drugs.

Basics about Depression

Depression has sometimes been described as "the common cold of mental illness." At any time, 13 to 20 percent of us have at least some degree of it.

Major depression and dysthymia—the two main classifications of depression—differ according to how chronic, severe, and long lasting they are. Major depression, which isn't too common, is characterized by a sharp contrast to usual functioning. A happy person can go along with his normal life and then, over a period of several days or weeks, can rapidly develop severe symptoms of depression. Dysthymia, on the other hand, is a chronic depression of low to moderate severity that lasts many months or years. It can hang like a pall over people's lives for years and years, eroding confidence and initiative and greatly diminishing joys and pleasures that are experienced.

Whether major or minor or some other type, depression can also be described by its features or symptoms. For example, some depressions involve biological or environmental triggers. These include premenstrual, postnatal, and menopausal depressions and seasonal affective disorder, or SAD (winter depression).

Atypical features, another classifier or subtype, involve mood reactivity and at least two of the following: increased appetite and/or weight gain, unexplained profound tiredness and exhaustion, too much sleep, and excessive sensitivity to rejection. Percentage-wise, this cluster of symptoms is the largest subtype of depression.

The Disadvantages of Antidepressant Drugs

Several different types of drugs are used in treating the various forms of depression, but each one has troublesome side effects. Tricyclic antidepressants, for example, often cause lethargy and lead to weight gain. Selective serotonin reuptake inhibitors (SSRIs), a popular group of antidepressants including Prozac and Zoloft, can cause fuzzy thinking, nausea, diarrhea, headache, and sexual side effects. Some physicians have even attributed an increased incidence of suicide or violence in people who take certain SSRIs.

Monoamine oxidase inhibitors (MAOIs) are so problematic that most psychiatrists no longer recommend them. The use of these drugs requires a number of strict dietary restrictions and special precautions (such as avoiding certain other drugs). If these precautions aren't followed, patients can develop a dangerous side effect—a severe hypertensive crisis. People who take MAOIs are instructed to carry an antidote and rush to the nearest emergency room if a severe, throbbing headache develops.

Clearly, natural treatments that work well for depression but don't have adverse side effects are desirable to many of the standard antidepressant drug treatments. Supplemental chromium appears to be one such natural treatment: it's been found to both boost the action of SSRI antidepressants and act as an antidepressant in its own right.

The Fascinating Way Chromium's Effects Were Discovered

The discovery of chromium's beneficial effects on depression began in a serendipitous way. One day, a longtime depressed patient of Malcolm McLeod, M.D., of Chapel Hill, North Carolina, told the psychiatrist that he had experienced dramatic improvements in his condition after taking a multivitamin and mineral supplement. McLeod was skeptical of supplements, so he subjected the patient's pills to scientific scrutiny.

After studying the supplement label, McLeod asked his patient to stop taking the supplement and participate in an experiment. McLeod gave the patient only one of the supplement's individual ingredients for an entire week; then he switched to a different individual ingredient the next week. The patient didn't know which of the individual supplements he was taking.

During the first, third, fourth, and fifth weeks of the experiment, the patient didn't feel any improvement and, in some cases, felt worse. During the second week, however, he felt a dramatic and immediate relief in his depression, along with other beneficial health effects, such as a decrease in appetite and an increase in energy.

At the end of the fifth week, the patient insisted on knowing what he took during the second week. He was told it was chromium picolinate. On his own initiative, the patient began to take 400 mcg of chromium daily from chromium picolinate. His sleep improved, his thinking became clearer, he lost his cravings for food and alcohol, and he became hopeful about the future. His depression cleared so completely that he eventually stopped taking the SSRI drug he had been taking.

McLeod's Discovery of Chromium's Beneficial Effects in Others

Amazed by the effects supplemental chromium had on this one patient, McLeod tried the experiment on several more patients with different symptoms. He got similar results. The difference in some of his patients after taking chromium supplements was so dramatic that McLeod had no choice but to believe he was on to something.

He applied for patents on the use of chromium for treating depression and premenstrual syndrome (PMS). He also published the results of his experiment in the April 1999 issue of the *Journal of Clinical Psychiatry*.

Then he began hearing from other psychiatrists—from around the United States and even from Australia and Sweden—who had witnessed similar positive effects from supplemental chromium in their practices. They told him that in some cases, supplemental chromium was life transforming for several of their patients.

McLeod also oversaw two more studies that found chromium supplementation helpful for many types of depression—as well as for premenstrual syndrome. And other researchers at the University of North Carolina and Duke University are now following up on his work: they're currently conducting studies of their own to try to verify his findings.

Chromium's Antidepressant Action

McLeod's first scientific paper—the write-up of his initial experiments—showed that chromium supplementation led to remission of longstanding, minor to moderate depression (dysthymia) in patients who were taking SSRI drugs. The SSRIs by themselves didn't eradicate these patients' depression, but when the patients took chromium supplements along with the SSRIs, their depression dramatically lifted and so did the side effects, such as fuzzy thinking, that they were having from taking the SSRIs.

Chromium supplementation, therefore, potentiated the action of the antidepressants and reduced the side effects of antidepressants. McLeod at first thought that's all chromium did. However, experiments with other patients confirmed that chromium supplementation all by itself acts as an antidepressant and is sometimes all that is needed to eradicate depression.

A few examples: one patient who had bipolar disorder and major depression had developed unacceptable side effects from several antidepressants. Lithium treatment caused a feeling of being slowed down and a thirty-pound weight gain. After starting to take chromium supplements, the patient was able to stop taking lithium and continue with chromium alone. He felt increasingly relaxed and stable and gradually lost twenty-three pounds. Other patients who couldn't take anti - depressant drugs because of undesirable side effects, such as loss of interest in sex, had their depression completely go away when they took chromium supplements.

How Chromium Might Work

Based on clinical evidence, McLeod and his colleagues at the University of North Carolina department of psychiatry have a few ideas about how chromium might work in the body to alleviate depression. As a potentiator of insulin, chromium allows blood sugar to enter brain cells more easily. Blood sugar is a primary fuel the brain needs to make chemical messengers that regulate mood and help us think clearly.

Chromium may also help facilitate the entry of tryptophan, an amino acid, into the brain. Tryptophan serves as an essential building block for chemical messengers, such as serotonin, which regulate mood, emotions, sleep, and appetite. Low levels of serotonin or dysfunctions of serotonin activity are associated with depression. Chromium may also enhance the release of stored chemical messengers, such as norepinephrine, that help promote normal mood functioning.

Serotonin
A neurotransmitter that regulates mood, emotions, sleep, and appetite. Disorders of serotonin activity are thought to be involved in depression.

It's interesting to note that depression is often associated with insulin resistance and poor utilization of blood sugar. Several studies show that type II diabetics are at increased risk for depression. Chromium of course improves insulin sensitivity and helps reverse type II diabetes—and many type II diabetics who take chromium supplements often report improvements in mood. By improving insulin sensitivity, chromium probably facilitates serotonin activity in the brain, thereby exerting some antidepressant effects.

The Type of Depression Chromium Seems to Help

Depression is a complex disorder; it should be emphasized that chromium isn't a cure-all for all types of depression. However, the more McLeod investigates the effect of chromium supplementation on depression, the more he suspects that it's helpful for people who have what psychiatrists call "depression with atypical features." These features, you'll recall, include cravings for sugar and carbohydrates, weight problems, lethargy, excess sleepiness, and excessive sensitivity to rejection by others.

The term "atypical" is something of a misnomer because about 40 percent of depressed people have these features. People with atypical symptoms usually don't receive effective treatment. They typically don't respond to common antidepressants, and MAIOs, which have been used as a treatment, have such dangerous side effects that most doctors don't want to use them.

Atypical Features

A term that classifies depression with symptoms including sugar cravings, overweight, lethargy, sleepiness, and sensitivity to rejection.

The good news is chromium supplementation seems to be particularly helpful for treating people with this subtype of depression. However, some depressed people without atypical symptoms also have responded to chromium supplements. Researchers need more time and study to determine all the different types of depressed people who respond favorably to chromium supplementation.

Chromium Is Also Helpful for PMS and Painful Periods

Some of McLeod's depressed female patients also suffered from premenstrual syndrome—characterized by such symptoms as mood swings, increased irritability or anxiety, carbohydrate cravings, over-eating, marked lack of energy, and sleep disturbances during the last week or several days before menstrual periods. Other female patients had painful periods with menstrual cramps. Upon receiving chromium supplements, their PMS symptoms and painful periods were alleviated.

In some women with severe PMS, chromium taken in combination with standard SSRI antidepressants totally eradicated their symptoms. In other women, chromium alone was all that was needed.

Most of these experiments were done under single-blind conditions—when the doctor knows what the patient is taking but the patient does not. However, one small pilot study that involved six women was a double-blind, placebo-controlled study—in other words, neither the doctor nor the patient knew what the patient was taking. This study found similar results: chromium augments the effects of standard antidepressants when needed. Some women got such marked relief that they made comments like "Without a doubt, that's the easiest period I've had in years" and "When my period started, I was completely surprised. I had none of the usual, difficult warning symptoms."

Chromium Might Alleviate Seasonal Blues

Some of McLeod's patients with seasonal affective disorder (SAD) also have been helped by chromium supplementation. Technically, SAD can mean recurrent mood swings during a particular season. However, it most often refers to recurrent depression during the fall and winter, when the daylight hours are shorter. Symptoms of this type of SAD include depressed mood, difficulty concentrating, excess sleep, decreased energy, increased appetite, and carbohydrate cravings—symptoms very much like those in depression with atypical features.

Recent research has found that mood swings during the winter months are common in healthy people. These people don't technically have SAD, but they feel slightly down, sadder, more irritable, or worry more during winter than they do during other times of year.

Simple treatments—such as getting more sun exposure, increasing physical activity, and making dietary changes—have been recommended for the seasonal blues. Taking chromium supplements seems like another good strategy because it has already proven helpful for some people with SAD.

I believe another reason for the winter blues is that many people eat more chromium-depleting sugar and refined grains during the winter holidays, especially from Halloween through New Year's Day. An increase in the intake of refined carbohydrates lowers chromium levels, probably inducing chromium deficiencies and subsequent winter blues in many people, escalating their need for chromium supplements.

Common Threads in Disorders Helped by Chromium

It may seem unbelievable that chromium could be effective for so many different mood disorders—depression, premenstrual syndrome, and winter blues. But researchers have noted that these disorders often share common symptoms—such as carbohydrate cravings and lethargy.

In addition, all of these disorders have responded to antidepressant medicines that increase brain levels of serotonin. This suggests that these disorders are closely related and are associated with low serotonin levels. Since chromium improves insulin sensitivity and probably, as a result, increases serotonin levels in the brain, supplemental chromium may prove to remedy a key factor in these conditions.

Chromium Is Worth Trying for Depression and PMS

Supplemental chromium is probably worth a try if a person has any of these disorders and hasn't responded to other treatments. Chromium is a very safe supplement, and most people are lacking in chromium and can benefit from supplements.

There have been few side effects reported in studies with depressed people, and those that have occurred have been mild. Some people report having vivid dreams (but not nightmares)—an effect which usually subsides after a few weeks.

Some people also report that if chromium is taken too late in the day, it may interfere with falling asleep. This effect can be counteracted by simply taking chromium earlier in the day, at least eight hours before bedtime. When taken early in the day, chromium tends to have an energizing effect for the first six hours or so and then seems to regulate sleep and reduce insomnia, according to McLeod.

Chromium doesn't seem to negatively interact with any medications. But chromium taken with excessive amounts of caffeine may cause some people to feel wired, so this combination is best avoided. Also, for reasons that aren't understood, a few patients who have taken chromium while also taking the popular antidepressant herb, St. John's wort, found that the combination worsened their depression and PMS. Therefore, it's probably best not to take chromium and St. John's wort at the same.

Chromium can make SSRI medications more effective and reduce the side effects they cause. If you currently take an SSRI or any other psychiatric drug and want to try chromium supplements, it's best to talk with your healthcare provider.

Chromium—A Natural Antidepressant

Chromium is an essential nutrient our bodies need on a daily basis to maintain blood sugar balance and insulin sensitivity. By boosting these actions, supplemental chromium acts as a natural antidepressant.

Consider that chromium supplements act faster than antidepressants, usually showing beneficial effects within a few days, rather than at least a month for antidepressants. Chromium supplements also have no serious side effects and are 20 to 50 times less expensive than antidepressant drugs. Considering all the evidence so far, chromium supplements probably should be the first choice for the treatment of mood disorders, before antidepressant drugs.

CHAPTER 7

OTHER BENEFITS AND AREAS FOR FUTURE RESEARCH

Chromium's beneficial effects on diabetes, Syndrome X, cholesterol problems, overweight, aging, depression, and PMS are very impressive. But this mineral has even more benefits, as well as potential benefits yet to be researched. For starters, supplemental chromium helps prevent osteoporosis. There's also evidence to suggest that chromium may be helpful for conditions as varied as acne, alcoholism, bulimia, nearsighted vision, and a common cause of female infertility. This chapter will fill you in on all the latest thinking of future areas of research for chromium supplementation.

Chromium Improves DHEA Levels and Helps Prevent Osteoporosis

In 1996, the results of an innovative study led by Gary Evans, Ph.D., was published in the *FASEB Journal*. Unfortunately, as is often the case, health writers and researchers missed the boat on how significant this research actually was.

At the time, it was known that insulin resistance interfered with calcium absorption into bone and led to high insulin levels, which markedly reduce the production of the antiaging, feel-good hormone DHEA. Evans also learned that postmenopausal women who had high insulin levels had low levels of DHEA. He wondered if chromium supplementation would reduce insulin levels and raise DHEA levels and therefore improve bone health in these women.

To put this idea to a test, Evans had twenty-seven postmenopausal women, ages fifty-two to sixty-three, take two capsules per day that contained either a placebo or 200 mcg of chromium as chromium picolinate for two months. For three months after that, no supplement was given; then the women were given the opposite supplement. The results that occurred during the period of chromium supplementation were impressive. Blood insulin levels dropped 38 percent, blood sugar levels decreased 26 percent, and DHEA levels increased 24 percent. In addition, the amount of calcium the women excreted decreased by half, and two key indicators of bone breakdown—the urinary hydroxyproline/creatinine ratio and the urinary calcium/creatinine ratio—decreased by about 20 percent.

This study showed that supplementing with chromium picolinate can go a long way toward preventing osteoporosis, especially in people who have insulin resistance—in other words, most people who are overweight, people who have Syndrome X or type II diabetes, and one-quarter of the thin population. Essentially, efficient insulin activity builds bone; inefficient insulin activity breaks down bone.

Osteoporosis
The condition of age-related bone loss in which the bones are more likely to break. More than 10 million women have this condition.

Chromium Boosts Postmenopausal Women's Estrogen Levels

Another key finding of this study was after taking chromium supplements for one month, the postmenopausal women's estrogen (estradiol) and DHEA (which can be converted to estrogen and other sex hormones) increased to levels resembling those of women in their thirties. Chromium supplements, therefore, can turn back the hormonal clock, perhaps delaying menopause and possibly reducing the adverse symptoms caused by the dramatic loss of hormones that typically occurs during menopause.

Osteoporosis and difficult menopauses are treated with estrogen by many doctors. However, estrogen is not an ideal treatment because it has been shown to increase the risk of certain types of cancer. This study suggested there is a natural way to increase estrogen levels in the body without actually taking estrogen: that is, to take chromium supplements. It seems that when insulin is functioning efficiently in the body, it keeps other hormones functioning more efficiently, too. Controlling insulin levels seems to be an effective way to hold back, delay, or improve age-related conditions, including osteoporosis and menopause.

The Chromium Connection to Alcoholism and Bulimia

In the last chapter, you learned that depression, premenstrual syndrome, and seasonal affective disorder all share a common link: low levels of serotonin or inefficient serotonin activity in the brain. Two other disorders, alcoholism and bulimia nervosa (bulimia, for short) share that same link. Chromium supplementation seems to enhance serotonin activity in the brain, and there's evidence to suggest that it may be helpful as an aid in the treatment of alcoholism and bulimia, just as it is for depression, premenstrual syndrome, and seasonal affective disorder.

Alcoholism is characterized by a tendency to drink excessively, unsuccessful attempts at stopping drinking, and continuing to drink despite adverse social, occupational, and health consequences. Bulimia is characterized by repeated episodes of binge eating (usually of sweets and grain-based foods), followed by purging (self-induced vomiting or taking laxatives or diuretics), or excessive exercise to counteract the effects of bingeing. Like alcoholics, bulimics have trouble stopping their behavior even when they understand that it is unhealthy for them.

Uncontrollable cravings (for alcohol or carbohydrates, probably stemming from disordered serotonin metabolism) seem to drive people to drink or eat excessively. Chromium supplementation diminishes cravings for sweets and carbohydrates, and it was reported to diminish cravings for alcohol in some of McLeod's depressed patients with frequent alcohol cravings. One of McLeod's patients who benefited had a family history of alcoholism.

Nutritionally oriented physicians have long believed that blood sugar imbalances lie at the core of alcoholism. Chromium, which acts as a blood sugar regulator, should therefore be helpful. My limited experience counseling people with bulimia leads me to believe that chromium is helpful for some of them, too.

A Success Story of One Woman Overcoming Bulimia

One of my clients—I'll call her Hope—had bulimia, depression, and Syndrome X (with high cholesterol, high triglycerides, and abdominal obesity). She was taking an SSRI antidepressant for the bulimia and depression, but it didn't seem to help much. Hope typically made herself vomit twice a day, even though she knew she shouldn't. She contacted me because she knew I specialized in the nutritional treatment of Syndrome X.

The standard nutrition-oriented approach would be to ignore the fact that she had Syndrome X and treat her eating disorder first. But I got the sense that disturbed blood sugar metabolism was at the crux of her problems. It seemed to cause her nearly uncontrollable cravings for carbohydrates, which prompted her to binge on carbohydrates, which in turn led her to induce vomiting because she felt so uncomfortably full.

I put her on an Anti-X program, which included a sugar-free, grain-free diet and a number of supplements, including chromium. It worked like a charm: she stopped bingeing, so she stopped purging, and conquered her longstanding battle with bulimia. She also felt brighter spirited and gradually started to lose weight and have her cholesterol and triglyceride levels come down.

It's hard to say whether it was the diet, the chromium supplements, or some of the other supplements (such as liquid zinc sulfate) that worked so effectively. I believe the whole program worked together to improve her inefficient insulin sensitivity and the numerous conditions that stemmed from that.

However, Hope is certain that chromium played an important role. A few times she forgot to take her chromium supplements and her cravings for carbohydrates came back with a vengeance, making it much more difficult for her to stay on her nutrition program.

Both bulimia and alcoholism are complex mind-body disorders with numerous factors that are probably involved. The story of Hope is not meant to indicate that chromium supplementation is effective for all cases of bulimia—only that it has proven tremendously helpful in some cases. The clinical and theoretical evidence suggesting beneficial effects from chromium supplementation for bulimia and alcoholism is so intriguing that both conditions should be future areas of research.

The Growing List of Conditions Associated with High Insulin

In Chapters 2 and 3, you learned that insulin resistance and high insulin levels can lead to the development of type II diabetes and cardiovascular disease, two of the most common diseases of aging. In Chapter 5, you learned that high insulin levels accelerate aging all throughout the body.

It shouldn't be surprising, then, that high insulin levels are associated with other diseases of aging. Several studies have established insulin resistance and high insulin levels as factors in cognitive disorders, impaired thinking processes, dementia, and even Alzheimer's disease. There is also substantial evidence that elevated levels of insulin increase the risk of breast, prostate, and colorectal cancers. Consider that type II diabetics have an increased risk of developing all three cancers.

The list of insulin-related disorders and disease processes keeps growing. Colorado State University health science researcher Loren Cordain, Ph.D., for example, has recently explained that the high insulin levels that go hand in hand with insulin resistance cause a cascade of hormonal shifts that favor unregulated cell growth in a variety of tissues. This unregulated cell growth may lead not only to breast, prostate, and colon cancers, but also to—believe it or not—acne, nearsightedness, and a female-specific condition called polycystic ovary syndrome. Reversing insulin resistance and reducing high insulin levels should nip these problems in the bud. Chromium supplementation, as you've learned, reverses insulin resistance and lowers insulin levels.

At first, the idea of chromium helping these varied conditions may seem farfetched. The insulin connection to these conditions is so new that, unfortunately, no research evaluating the effectiveness of chromium supplementation in these conditions has been conducted. But clinical and theoretical evidence suggests therapeutic value from supplemental chromium, so future studies are warranted.

The Chromium Connection to Acne

As early as 1940, research suggested that acne is a result of impaired sugar metabolism or insulin resistance of the skin. To measure the ability of the body to handle sugar, glucose tolerance tests have been performed on acne patients. Blood sugar levels during glucose tolerance tests seem to be normal in acne patients, but repetitive skin biopsies reveal their skin's glucose tolerance is significantly impaired. Considering this evidence, one researcher coined the term "skin diabetes" to describe the disorder of acne.

Chromium regulates blood sugar levels and improves insulin sensitivity. Insulin promotes the uptake of blood sugar by the cells, including skin cells. When insulin is functioning efficiently, improved glucose tolerance results throughout the body, including the skin.

As another line of thinking, consider that teenaged boys who eat many junk foods and drink a lot of soft drinks are the group of people most likely to develop acne. Sweets and white-flour products, such as pizza, pasta, and bread, are deficient in chromium, and soft drinks are totally void of chromium. Furthermore, sweets, white-flour products, and soft drinks promote losses of chromium from the body. It's very possible that low chromium levels are a factor in the development of acne.

In one study from nearly twenty years ago, high-chromium yeast was reported to produce rapid improvements in patients with acne. Unfortunately, no one has followed up on that research yet. Nevertheless, most Americans (and teenagers in particular) are lacking chromium in their diets, so chromium supplementation, together with avoiding sugar and refined grains, seems like a worthwhile nutrition strategy.

High-chromium yeast can be problematic, so I would recommend a better-tolerated source of chromium, such as chromium picolinate. Many people have hidden yeast sensitivities or a tendency to develop yeast infections and do best avoiding daily supplements of yeast.

The Chromium Connection to Nearsightedness

The idea that chromium supplementation might help prevent or delay the development of nearsightedness may seem harder to believe than anything else discussed here. However, keep in mind that research over the last decade or so

Nearsightedness
Difficulty seeing things at a distance. Poor nutrition, including lack of chromium, plays a role in its development.

has proven that optimal levels of nutrients are critical for protecting eye health and vision.

First, some basics: Nearsightedness may be partly genetic in origin, but it is also attributed to the extra strain industrialized people put on their eyes by constantly reading or performing near-visual tasks during the growing years. Poor nutrition, especially a high intake of chromium-depleting refined carbohydrates, plays a contributing role.

Benjamin Lane, O.D., C.N.S., an optometrist, nutritionist, and researcher from Lake Hiawatha, New Jersey, discovered the chromium connection to nearsightedness in the early 1980s. He evaluated the results of 120 consecutive nutrition workups from his files and reported his results in the *Journal of the International Academy of Preventive Medi-*

cine: chromium deficiency is strongly tied to the development and progression of nearsightedness.

Chromium is needed for the proper function of all muscles, but the muscles that we use more today than ever before are the ciliary muscles, the muscles that help the eyes focus so we can read. If there isn't enough chromium in our bloodstream, then long, sustained eye focusing cannot be maintained.

Many children eat tremendous amounts of chromium-depleting sugar and white-flour products, but they don't develop nearsightedness until their chromium reserves run out. As soon as they lose their chromium reserves, they rapidly develop nearsightedness under that stress of eye focusing, according to Lane.

Avoiding chromium-depleting, blood–sugar-raising, refined carbohydrates is one of the best nutritional strategies to try to prevent the development or progression of nearsightedness. But many people continue to eat these foods. In addition, Lane believes some people have inborn chromium deficiency. So, chromium supplementation may be needed for extra protection against nearsightedness. With our society doing more near-visual work than ever before, this is an important area for future research.

Polycystic Ovary Syndrome— A Newly Recognized Condition

Polycystic ovary syndrome (PCOS) is a newly recognized condition associated with insulin resistance and high insulin levels. It's characterized by symptoms such as ovarian cysts, irregular menstrual periods, elevated levels of male sex hormones such as testosterone, excess facial hair, acne, and often obesity. The most common cause of infertility among women in the United States, this disorder involves a woman's eggs maturing in the ovary but not being released.

Studies have shown that high insulin levels stimulate the production of male sex hormones by the ovaries and may impede ovulation and contribute to infertility. High levels of insulin, as you may recall, affect the balance of other hormones in the body.

Polycystic Ovary Syndrome
An insulin-related condition that affects females, causing ovarian cysts, irregular menstrual periods, excess facial hair, and sometimes infertility.

Like Syndrome X, PCOS increases the risk of other serious diseases associated with insulin resistance, such as type II diabetes. Virtually no nutritional research has been done on this condition, but improving insulin sensitivity has become established as a baseline treatment strategy in PCOS. In addition, improvements in PCOS have been reported by some women who have followed an Anti-X-type program that included chromium supplementation. Since chromium supplementation has fewer side effects than insulin-sensitizing drugs, its effectiveness in PCOS should be pursued in clinical trials.

Other Insulin-Related Conditions

There are several lines of research to suggest that sleep apnea and some types of iron overload may result from, or be aggravated by, insulin resistance and high insulin levels—and may, therefore, benefit from chromium supplementation.

Sleep apnea is a potentially fatal disorder of a breathing disruption during sleep. Loud snoring, gasping sounds, and disordered breathing during sleep are common symptoms. People who have abdominal obesity and type II diabetes are most apt to develop this problem. I have not had any clients diagnosed with sleep apnea, but I have had a number of Syndrome X clients who have reported that their snoring dramatically decreased after following an Anti-X program. McLeod has also reported that chromium supplementation can improve sleep disturbances. Since sleep apnea is such a serious disorder, investigating whether chromium supplementation could improve this condition seems like an area worth pursuing.

Iron overload is a storage of excess iron in organs such as the liver. There is hereditary iron overload (called hereditary hemachromatosis), and there is also insulin–resistance-associated iron overload. In one study, 94 percent of people with unexplained iron overload in the liver had Syndrome X.

The standard treatment for both types of iron overload is to have blood drawn regularly to reduce iron levels in the body. However, chromium supplementation may also be helpful. Many people with iron overload have reduced insulin sensitivity, and iron is antagonistic to chromium. Excess iron, therefore, may be displacing chromium, causing chromium deficiency; so supplemental chromium (in addition to blood draws) may be therapeutic.

The web of diseases and abnormalities associated with insulin resistance and high insulin levels seems to be far reaching and complex. Researchers will likely be investigating all the insulin connections to various ailments for decades. In the meantime, before all the research is conducted, you should become savvy to protect your health. If you learn that poor insulin function may be involved in the development of a condition you have or are prone to, think about supplemental chromium as a possible remedy that may be helpful.

CHAPTER 8

How to Buy and Use Chromium

By now, you've read about the impressive health benefits of chromium and learned that taking chromium supplements is one of the best things you can do to protect yourself from the blood–sugar- and insulin-related health problems that run rampant in our society. You're probably ready to learn more about how to supplement with chromium. This chapter will answer what you need to know about chromium supplements, so you can make the most educated decisions about to how to use chromium for your best health.

Who Should Take Chromium Supplements?

From my experience counseling clients, virtually everyone can benefit from supplemental chromium. Most Americans have grown up on a diet containing chromium-depleting sugar and white-flour products, which gradually leads to at least marginal chromium deficiencies. This is why blood sugar highs and lows and conditions such as overweight, Syndrome X, and type II diabetes are so common today.

The best way to know if you need chromium supplements is to consult a nutritionist or nutrition-oriented health professional who can evaluate your individual intake, needs, and symptoms. The second best way is the try-it-and-see approach: Try chromium supplements for a month or two and see if you experience beneficial effects on your health. Look for improvements in energy, mood, weight control, sugar cravings, or heart disease risk factors. The more you need chromium, the more you'll respond to supplementation. Some people with depression respond within a day or two.

Even if you are healthy (not overweight and not at risk for diabetes or heart disease), a small dose of supplemental chromium—say, 100–200 mcg—is recommended to insure that you meet your daily needs. As you'll remember, 90 percent of Americans don't meet the minimum suggested safe and adequate daily intake for chromium of 50 mcg. Over the long run, this puts people at risk for many health problems. Fortunately, a deficiency can be prevented with daily chromium supplements.

The Different Forms of Chromium Supplements

There are many different types of chromium supplements. Most people don't have any idea which one they should choose. The terms can get a bit confusing, so here are the basics:

GTF refers to glucose tolerance factor, the term originally given to an active form of chromium that researchers found affected blood sugar control. This active form of chromium was isolated from yeast and was better utilized by animals than chromium chloride, one of the earliest chromium compounds—an inorganic compound of chromium combined with chloride. The active form isolated from yeast is sometimes called yeast GTF.

Some researchers proposed a possible composition for GTF, but it was never shown that this specific composition existed. While GTF is sometimes still found in supplements, the term GTF is outdated and not used by many researchers today.

Chromium polynicotinate, a type of chromium supplement now out on the market, is a mixture of nicotinate (a form of vitamin B_3) and chromium combined with water. There's been a lot of hype about this form, but it has not proven to be absorbed well by the body.

Several organic compounds of chromium—compounds that contain carbon—are on the market. The different forms are compounds of chromium combined or chelated with various amino acids or organic acids in an effort to facilitate chromium absorption. To give you a few examples, chromium picolinate is chromium combined or chelated with picolinic acid; chromium arginate is chromium combined with arginine; chromium aspartate is chromium combined with aspartic acid; and chromium citrite is chromium combined with citric acid. Most of these forms, other than chromium picolinate, have not been extensively studied.

Chelator
A chemical or carrier protein that combines with a mineral and aids in moving it into the bloodstream and throughout the body.

Speaking a bit more scientifically, the minerals we need in our bodies are electrically charged. They have to be de-energized before they can approach and enter the body's cells. This can be done if they're attached to special chemical substances called chelators. Gary Evans, Ph.D., a USDA researcher, discovered picolinate to be a superior chelator and showed that it very effectively cloaks the charge of chromium so it can be carried by the blood to the cells that need it. Chromium picolinate is the most researched form of chromium. Numerous studies have found it's the best absorbed and best utilized form of chromium on the market.

The Safety of Chromium Supplements

If you're concerned about the safety of taking chromium, don't be. Nutritional chromium, the form of chromium found in foods and nutritional supplements, is considered one of the safest mineral nutrients. In animal experiments, chromium has demonstrated a lack of toxicity at extremely high levels—levels several thousand times the estimated safe and adequate daily dietary intake (ESADDI) limit of 200 mcg per day. There is no evidence of toxic effects or widespread health problems related to chromium supplementation in humans or in animals.

Unfortunately, in 1995, a controversial study was conducted, and some people got the idea that chromium picolinate could cause cancer. In the study, chromium picolinate caused chromosome damage in hamster ovarian cells in test-tube experiments. This result wasn't particularly surprising: the amount of chromium that was applied directly to these cells was 3,000 times the blood level of people who take chromium picolinate supplements. Very few essential minerals tested in this way would pass.

The standard test for determining whether chemicals cause cancer is the Ames test—an experiment in which a chemical is added to five different types of bacteria that reproduce rapidly and show adverse changes in their offspring. Chromium picolinate has been independently tested using the Ames test and has passed with flying colors.

The real test is not so much what happens in test-tube experiments but what happens in human and animal experiments. Chromium picolinate has been found to be extraordinarily safe in human and animal studies, and it certainly hasn't caused cancer. Its effects have been therapeutic, not toxic. As one example, remember that rats whose diets were supplemented with chromium picolinate lived 37 percent longer than rats who didn't receive supplemental chromium. Chromium supplements are safe: the far greater risk to health is not to take chromium supplements than to take them.

Side Effects from Chromium Are Rare

Most people do not experience any side effects from taking chromium. The side effects that have been reported have been few and minor, such as slight rashes or dizziness. If you experience symptoms such as these, try switching to a different form of chromium. Several of McLeod's depressed patients experienced dizzy spells while taking chromium polynicotinate but didn't have this symptom when they took chromium picolinate.

A few other side effects that McLeod has noticed from his research are increased and vivid dreaming after beginning chromium supplementation (which usually subsides after a few weeks) and a tendency to have trouble falling asleep if chromium is taken too close to bedtime. Trouble falling asleep can easily be avoided by taking chromium early in the day.

Also, a few people have developed headaches *after* discontinuing chromium. This symptom generally is considered to be a sign of glucose tolerance problems. When these people started taking chromium supplements again, their headaches disappeared.

Choosing a High-Quality Supplement

Choosing a chromium supplement isn't as simple as walking into a store and grabbing any supplement that says chromium. To get the most value for the money you spend, there are several tricks of the trade.

First, avoid brand-name supplements sold in drugstores and supermarkets, and look instead for one of the quality brands sold in health food stores and natural food supermarkets. Commercial brands often contain artificial colors (for example, blue, red, or yellow dyes), hidden forms of sugar (for example, maltodextrin), mineral oil, and long lists of unrecognizable words that are usually unnecessary excipients, binders, and fillers. Health food brands usually don't have these ingredients: They may be slightly more expensive, but you get better value in terms of quality.

Second, when choosing between capsules and tablets, keep in mind that capsules tend to be "cleaner"—in other words, they usually have fewer undesirable fillers than tablets. I also usually recommend capsules over tablets because capsules tend to be easier for the body to break down and easier for people to swallow.

Third, read labels carefully and look for the amount of elemental, or pure, chromium a supplement supplies. Chromium comes in different forms (chromium picolinate, chromium aspartate, chromium chelate, and so on), and each one of these forms supplies a different amount of elemental chromium. The amount of chromium compound that the supplement supplies is not important, but the amount of *elemental* chromium is.

This used to be a bit confusing for consumers, but supplement labels now should list the amount of elemental chromium in a standardized way—stating, for example, "200 mcg chromium (as chromium picolinate)" or "200 mcg elemental chromium (from chromium picolinate)." Either of these two listings means that the supplement supplies 200 mcg of elemental chromium from chromium picolinate.

Another way of finding a good chromium supplement is to look for the Chromax trademark in the Supplement Facts label on many supplements.

Chromax® chromium picolinate is the best-absorbed form, and the form that has proven most effective against insulin resistance. Therefore, it's the form that's worth seeking out.

Guidelines for How Much Chromium You Should Take

The amount of chromium a person needs depends upon age, overall health, diet, and stress and activity levels. Here are some guidelines:

- The amount of chromium considered safe and adequate for children seven years and older is 50–200 mcg. However, health conditions such as diabetes increase those needs. If you're a parent planning supplementation for a child, it's always best to discuss supplementation with a nutritionally oriented professional.

- If you're an adult, 200 mcg daily should be sufficient for the general prevention of insulin resistance and all the adverse health conditions that result from it.

- If you have reactive hypoglycemia (blood sugar lows a while after eating sweets) or if you're mildly depressed and/or slightly overweight, 400 mcg daily seems to be more therapeutic.

- If you have any one of the conditions involved in Syndrome X—obesity, hypertension, unhealthy triglyceride levels or poor cholesterol profiles—or if these conditions run in your family—try 400–800 mcg daily. It's best to split the amount you take in two to three smaller doses during the day. This amount also can be helpful if you have strong cravings for sugar.

- If you have type II diabetes, 1,000 mcg daily is recommended. This recommendation, though, comes with a caveat: if you are taking medication to control your glucose, start with 200 mcg of chromium per day for a week and monitor your glucose levels closely. Continue to increase the amount of chromium you take by 200 mcg per week until you reach 1,000 mcg, and then have your physician adjust your medication accordingly. Supplemental chromium works so well at improving insulin function that less medication to control glucose usually is needed.

Finding the Dose That's Right for You

If you have health problems, determining the dose of chromium that's best for you sometimes takes a bit of experimenting. If you have sugar cravings, for example, you'll probably find 200 mcg helpful but not near as effective at controlling your symptoms and improving your condition as 400 mcg daily. Most people can experiment with daily doses between 100–400 mcg and evaluate how they feel to determine the dose that's best for them.

If you run into trouble figuring out how much chromium to take, or if you have a serious health problem, see a nutritionist or nutrition-oriented physician who can help you fine-tune your supplement program. A nutrition-minded health professional can evaluate your needs based on your diet, physical activity levels, symptoms, and medical history and may sometimes order hair analysis or other tests to better assess your chromium status and make recommendations of the doses that are best for you.

What Doctors Tend to Think about Chromium

Don't expect your physician to agree with your decision to take chromium or to be knowledgeable about the many ways supplemental chromium can help your health. As Nobel laureate Linus Pauling, Ph.D., once said, "If a doctor isn't 'up' on something, he's 'down' on it."

Most doctors and health educators haven't received much nutrition training and tend to dismiss nutritional treatments because they don't know much about them. Even if doctors or health educators are open to the idea of nutritional treatments, they often are so busy that they have a hard time staying up to date on the latest nutritional research.

The evidence pointing toward the use of chromium for conditions covered in this book is unmistakable (or, in the case of the conditions mentioned in Chapter 7, strongly suggestive). By reading this book, you probably know more now about chromium than your doctor does. Don't get frustrated by this. Just try to encourage your doctor to learn more. Share this book with him, pointing specifically to the scientific references in the Selected References section of this book. That way your doctor can look up the studies himself and see that the information written in this book is grounded in science. If your doctor seems unwilling to do this, switch to a doctor who is more willing to work with you or seek guidance from a nutrition-oriented health professional.

Choosing between Chromium in a Multiple and Chromium by Itself

Most multivitamin and mineral supplements contain chromium, so a natural question is whether you should take a multiple that contains chromium or a chromium supplement by itself. The answer to that question depends on your reasons for supplementing with chromium.

If you're healthy and simply want to stay healthy,

taking a multivitamin/mineral that contains chromium offers good assurance that you're covering the bases of your daily needs for chromium and other essential nutrients. However, many multivitamin/minerals that supply chromium use a form such as chromium chloride, which is the least effective type, or other types that haven't been properly researched. To get your money's worth and to make sure you're getting chromium in its most absorbable and usable form, look for a multiple (or diabetic or sports formula) that contains chromium from chromium picolinate. To do that, you usually have to read the fine print.

If you need supplemental chromium for therapeutic reasons—say, to help reverse insulin resistance—then taking separate chromium supplements along with a multivitamin and mineral supplement or other therapeutic supplements usually works best. For the layperson who wants to keep supplements simple, I often recommend starting with something like Alpha betic™ once-a-day formula by Abkit. It has 200 mcg of chromium (as chromium picolinate), along with other nutrients important for insulin function, such as alpha-lipoic acid (which you'll learn about in the next chapter). Therefore, it's a good base supplement for people with insulin resistance, such as those who are overweight or have Syndrome X or type II diabetes. However, type II diabetics and those with Syndrome X respond best to higher doses of chromium, so they should take extra chromium supplements to reach a total of between 600 and 1,000 mcg of supplemental chromium per day.

Advantages of Having Separate Chromium Supplements

Even if you take a multiple that supplies adequate chromium, it's a good idea to have separate supplements of 200 mcg of chromium on hand to take if you occasionally indulge in a sweet or white-flour product, such as white bread or pasta. This is unconventional nutrition advice, but it works well for most of my clients (as long as it's not taken to an extreme or taken too late in the day).

As a nutritionist, I must emphasize that one of the best things you can do for your health is to steer clear of nutrient-deficient refined sugars and grains as often as possible. The more you do this, the better your health will be. However, practically speaking, many people find it difficult to avoid these foods completely (especially during special occasions). At those times, it makes sense to supplement with chromium.

When refined carbohydrates are eaten, blood sugar levels rise and the body reacts by releasing insulin into the bloodstream to stimulate the uptake of blood sugar into the tissues. What most people don't know is that the body also signals the release of an active form of chromium from sites in the liver and other areas into the bloodstream to help insulin do its job. Once chromium is done being used this way, it is lost in the urine.

Eating refined carbohydrates, therefore, is a double-whammy for maintaining optimal chromium levels: these foods are deficient in chromium and eating these foods provokes chromium losses. For these reasons, you should try hard not to eat refined carbohydrates and should supplement with extra chromium if you do. Supplementing with chromium helps some of my clients have their cake and eat it, too, so they can enjoy special occasions without such severe nutritional consequences.

CHAPTER 9

NUTRIENTS AND OTHER FACTORS THAT ENHANCE CHROMIUM'S EFFECTS

As you've learned throughout this book, supplemental chromium works well all by itself to improve many different conditions. But chromium can work even better when you combine it with other synergistic nutrients, a good diet, stress reduction, and physical activity. This chapter gives you a rundown of the many factors that can help you get the most effectiveness out of the chromium you take so you can enjoy better overall health.

Chromium Works Best with Other Nutrients

The health benefits of chromium are impressive, but chromium is still just one nutrient. There are more than twenty other essential nutrients we need to keep our bodies functioning optimally. We shouldn't forget about our needs for other nutrients or our health will suffer.

Nutrients always work best when they're part of a balanced or targeted program designed specifically for the individual. This section will highlight some of the other nutrients you should think about to help chromium work best for the improvement or maintenance of your health.

Vitamins C and E

As you learned in Chapter 5, high blood sugar levels generate high levels of harmful free radicals that damage and age the body. Blood–sugar-related conditions such as Syndrome X and type II diabetes are characterized by excessive levels of free radicals and low levels of protective antioxidants. That's why these conditions are associated with accelerated aging.

Chromium is a natural for improving insulin function and thereby lowering blood sugar levels. But people with Syndrome X and type II diabetes can also benefit from supplementing their diets with antioxidants to squelch the excess free radicals that are produced, which contribute to the insulin resistance disease process.

The most important antioxidants are vitamin C, the key water-soluble antioxidant in the body, and vitamin E, the key fat-soluble antioxidant. These nutrients not only work synergistically to scavenge free radicals and reduce damage and aging in the body, they also play important roles in protection against cardiovascular disease. Vitamin C and vitamin E, therefore, are important nutrients for the public at large, but they're even more important for those with Syndrome X and type II diabetes who are much more prone to developing cardiovascular disease.

Just as most people don't get adequate levels of chromium in the diet, many people also don't get adequate levels of vitamins C and E from the diet. Supplements, therefore, are recommended, particularly for people with insulin–resistance-related conditions. Individual needs vary, but 500–2,000 mg of vitamin C and 400–800 IU of natural vitamin E are prudent doses for most people.

B Vitamins

The B vitamins include B_1 (thiamine), B_2 (riboflavin), B_3 (niacin and niacinamide), pantothenic acid (vitamin B_5), B_6 (pyridoxine), B_{12}, folic acid, biotin, choline, inositol, and PABA (para-aminobenzoic acid). Each B vitamin has its own unique roles and properties, but they often work together in the body and are commonly talked about together.

As a group, B vitamins help the body burn the food we eat efficiently, thereby helping to give us energy. They're often called "the antistress vitamins," because our need for B vitamins increases dramatically during times of stress. B vitamins have a well-documented role in maintaining a healthy nervous system, which has led many practitioners to use B-complex vitamins or individual B vitamins to alleviate psychiatric symptoms such as mild depression, anxiety, and nervousness.

Multi-ingredient supplements containing chromium picolinate and specific B vitamins found synergistic in alleviating depression or anxiety may one day be developed. In the meantime, many people who are under a lot of stress can benefit from taking a B-50 or B-100 complex (which supplies 50–100 mg of most of the major B vitamins) in addition to taking chromium supplements.

Minerals

There are more than a dozen essential minerals: each has critical roles in maintaining health. After chromium, the two most important for supporting optimal insulin function are zinc and magnesium. Zinc is needed to help the pancreas produce insulin, to allow insulin to work more effectively, and to protect insulin receptors on cells. Magnesium is needed for the production and release of insulin and to maintain insulin sensitivity. Therefore, while chromium is critical for preventing and reversing insulin resistance, so are zinc and magnesium. Doses of 30–50 mg of zinc and 400 mg of magnesium are often used in therapeutic programs for combating insulin resistance.

Many people can help meet their daily needs for minerals by taking well-rounded multiminerals or multivitamins/minerals. However, caution should be taken about supplementing with iron. Excessive amounts of iron can increase free radical activity in the body and are associated with insulin–resistance-related conditions. Iron may crowd chromium out from doing its job as an insulin potentiator. Therefore, unless a legitimate iron deficiency has been diagnosed, people should choose multimineral supplements without iron.

Essential Fatty Acids

Like chromium, omega-3 essential fatty acids help improve glucose tolerance and reverse insulin resistance. They also lower high blood pressure and high blood triglycerides and protect against heart disease.

Eating coldwater fish, omega-3-enriched eggs, flaxseeds, and dark green leafy vegetables boosts omega-3 intake adequately for the promotion of good health in many people. But some people, especially those with Syndrome X or those who don't eat fish, can benefit from taking 1–3 grams of EPA- and DHA-rich fish oil supplements daily. Diabetics, however, should work with a nutrition-savvy healthcare professional before they try omega-3 supplements.

Alpha-Lipoic Acid and Silymarin (Milk Thistle)

Alpha-lipoic acid, a vitaminlike substance, and silymarin, the active ingredient in the herb milk thistle, are not essential nutrients. But both are antioxidants that bolster liver function, lower blood glucose levels, and reverse insulin resistance.

In my nutritional practice, I have found that one

or both of these supplements work well with chromium supplements for countering Syndrome X and type II diabetes. Therapeutic doses range from 280–525 mg of standardized milk thistle extract daily and 100–600 mg of alpha-lipoic acid daily, depending on the severity of the condition.

A Picture of the Future— Chromium Nutrient Combinations

Right now, it's best to work with a knowledgeable health professional to take the many nutrient supplements that are available and develop a targeted nutrition program with chromium for the treatment of various conditions. But there's good news on the horizon for consumers.

Researchers are currently investigating different individual nutrients to find nutrients that help chromium work even better for the nutritional support of various systems and conditions. Areas of investigation include synergistic chromium-nutrient compounds for better blood sugar control, the normalization of cholesterol levels, maintenance of cardiovascular health, bone health support, and improved mood.

Two chromium-nutrient combinations seem especially promising right now. One is chromium picolinate plus conjugated linoleic acid (CLA), which is a fatty acid. In test-tube studies, the two ingredients together dramatically improved glucose uptake into human muscle cells, even without the presence of insulin! Researchers aren't quite sure how the ingredients are working without the action of insulin, but this finding is dramatic. It might mean that in the near future, chromium picolinate plus CLA could be used to promote better blood sugar control in type I diabetics who no longer produce adequate insulin.

The second chromium-nutrient compound worth keeping an eye out for is chromium picolinate plus niacin (vitamin B_3). Both chromium and niacin are known independently to lower high blood cholesterol levels. But niacin is usually needed in high doses of several grams a day to produce therapeutic effects. These doses often lead to side effects such as flushing—an uncomfortable tingling of the skin. Combining chromium picolinate with niacin seems to solve this problem. It allows much lower doses of niacin to be used for therapeutic benefits without side effects.

Some supplement manufacturing companies plan to make targeted chromium compound products like these available to consumers over the next several years. These products have the potential to make supplemental chromium even more therapeutic, so keep an eye out for them.

A New Product— Chromium plus Biotin

One targeted chromium compound has just recently become available. It's a combination of chromium picolinate plus biotin. It can be found under the trademark name Diachrome™—both on the supplement facts label and sometimes as the name of the product itself.

This product was developed after researchers tried to find nutrients that worked synergistically with chromium to improve sugar and fat metabolism. They investigated several different nutrients and found that biotin worked best with chromium for this purpose.

Chromium plus Biotin Improves Blood Sugar and Cholesterol

Studies conducted at the University of Vermont College of Medicine and the Chicago Center for Clinical Research have found that this combination leads to enhanced blood sugar control and improvements in cholesterol profiles. Here's a rundown of this recent research:

- In muscle cell culture studies, supplementation with chromium picolinate plus biotin enhanced blood sugar uptake four times more than supplementation with biotin or chromium picolinate alone.

- In studies with obese rats with high insulin levels—Syndrome X animal models—supplementation with chromium picolinate plus biotin (and chromium picolinate alone) improved rates of glucose disposal compared to the rats who received no chromium supplementation.

- In studies with type II diabetics who drank a high-carbohydrate, meal-replacement–type drink twice daily, fasting blood sugar levels and glycated hemoglobin levels skyrocketed in the diabetics who did not receive any chromium supplements. However, these levels did not significantly change in diabetics who took chromium picolinate plus biotin. This means that chromium picolinate plus biotin significantly controlled some of the negative effects of sugar intake in diabetics.

Therefore, chromium picolinate plus biotin is a combination that can help maintain and control healthy blood sugar levels, promote healthy fat metabolism, improve insulin sensitivity, and promote healthy cholesterol profiles. It's an exciting new nutrient combination that should be helpful for people with Syndrome X and type II diabetes.

A Multi-Ingredient Chromium Compound to Promote Weight Loss

A multi-ingredient product that enhances chromium's ability to promote weight and fat loss also has recently been developed. The patented combination of four ingredients is found in one new product called Metabolic Makeover, which is available exclusively through the QVC home shopping television channel and its website, www.qvc.com. You should be able to find similar products by other companies on store shelves in the near future.

The combination of ingredients to look for is chromium picolinate along with three other ingredients—carnitine, hydroxycitric acid (HCA), and biotin or pyruvate. Carnitine, often called an amino acid, is a nutrient that picks up fats and drops them off where the body burns them for fuel. HCA is a natural substance extracted primarily from the dried rind of the fruit of a South Asian plant, *Garcinia cambogia*. Pyruvate is a key compound needed for the body to produce energy.

The combination of these four ingredients have been found to have a "hepatothermic effect"—in other words, they enhance metabolism in the liver, which is important for enhancing weight loss.

A short pilot study involving sixteen primarily Samoan-American, obese people who weighed between 200 and 500 pounds showed that this combination is beneficial for weight loss. Supplementation with the four ingredients, together with a high-protein diet and moderate walking, led to dramatic results in three to four weeks. The people lost an average of three pounds of weight and five pounds of fat per week. The heaviest person actually lost twenty-six pounds of weight and fifty pounds of fat in twenty-four days! What's more, lean body mass increased and the supplement takers reported increased energy.

Improving Your Diet to Help Chromium Work Better

You can take chromium or chromium combination supplements regularly, but if you consistently eat a junk-food diet, the supplements aren't going to work very well. Chromium can improve blood sugar and insulin function, but eating foods that stress blood sugar and insulin function can negate many of chromium's positive effects.

Remember: insulin-resistance conditions such as overweight, Syndrome X, and type II diabetes are nutritional conditions. That means that diet plays an indispensable role in the reversal of these conditions.

If you're really serious about wanting to overcome insulin-related conditions, you should take chromium supplements *and* change your diet. This section will give you diet tips so you can enhance chromium's key role of improving insulin sensitivity and thereby lowering blood sugar and insulin levels.

Lower Your Carbohydrate Intake

Rule number one with diet is to avoid high-carbohydrate refined sugar and refined grains, those pesky ingredients that find their way into popular foods such as sweets, candy, bread, pasta, and snack foods, as well as soft drinks. Following this guideline can be difficult at first because refined carbohydrates are virtually everywhere in our modern society. However, when you go against the grain of social pressure to eat these foods, you go a long way toward improving blood sugar function and allowing the chromium you take to work more effectively at improving insulin function.

If you have severe blood sugar problems such as type II diabetes, it's best to avoid other high-carbohydrate foods such as whole grains, starchy vegetables like potatoes, and dried fruits. Although these foods are generally more nutritious than refined carbohydrates, they're not as good at promoting optimal blood sugar and insulin function as non-starchy vegetables—such as salad greens, spinach, broccoli, cabbage, cauliflower, green beans, and asparagus. By avoiding grains and other high-carbohydrate foods and eating non-starchy vegetables, carbohydrate intake is dramatically reduced. This helps lower blood sugar and insulin levels, giving you some of the benefits of calorie restriction that you learned about in Chapter 5. Together with chromium supplementation, a lower-carbohydrate diet works very well at reversing insulin resistance.

Get Adequate Protein and Fat

Getting adequate protein and fat also is important for eating a diet that works well with chromium supplementation. Protein stimulates the production of glucagon, a hormone that opposes insulin and is needed for the maintenance of a healthy metabolism and the building and repairing of muscles. If you take chromium but don't eat enough protein, metabolism can slow and muscle mass can be lost rather than be improved.

Getting adequate protein—and fat—also satisfies the appetite and makes it easier to stick to a lower-carbohydrate diet that can lower insulin levels. Although many people think all types of fat are unhealthy, that's simply not true. Reducing carbohydrate intake and eating more monounsaturated fats, such as olives, olive oil, avocado, and many nuts, improves insulin sensitivity. Emphasizing monounsaturated fats *and* omega-3 fats, such as those in coldwater fish, while avoiding other types of fat, is even better. Eating the right types of fat and avoiding the wrong ones adds to the effect of taking chromium supplements to improve insulin sensitivity.

Lastly, try adding a little spice to your diet. Laboratory experiments by USDA researchers have found that cinnamon, cloves, apple pie spice, bay leaves, and turmeric potentiate insulin activity more than threefold. Using these flavorful additions to your cooking is another way to keep insulin working effectively, along with the help of supplemental chromium.

The Importance of Stress Reduction, Adequate Sleep, and Exercise

Many people don't realize it, but lifestyle factors, such as excessive stress, lack of sleep, and lack of physical activity, contribute to the development of insulin resistance. Addressing these factors can only add to the effects of taking chromium supplements to improve insulin sensitivity.

Excessive stress interferes with efforts to improve insulin sensitivity. It raises levels of cortisol, and chronic elevations of cortisol lead to increased insulin levels, diminished muscle use of blood sugar for energy, and lower levels of the antiaging hormone DHEA.

Stress reduction through various means helps promote health and youthful body function because it raises DHEA levels. You learned in Chapters 5 and 7 that taking chromium picolinate supplements also raises DHEA levels (in addition to lowering insulin levels). So the combination of chromium supplementation and reducing stress is likely to be extra effective at holding back aging.

People who sleep seven and a half to eight and

a half hours a night process carbohydrates more efficiently than those who sleep less. People who deprive themselves of sleep, on the other hand, are on the fast track to developing insulin resistance. Getting adequate sleep, therefore, is another effective strategy to avoid sabotaging the beneficial effects of chromium on insulin sensitivity.

Physical activity increases insulin sensitivity, helps build muscle, and reduces stress, not to mention that it significantly reduces the risk of cardiovascular disease and type II diabetes. Many people actually can reverse insulin resistance with diet and chromium and other supplements, but some people need the extra benefits of regular physical activity. If you start an exercise program, keep in mind that strenuous exercise increases chromium losses from the body, so chromium supplementation is more important than ever.

CONCLUSION

Chromium is an essential mineral needed in tiny amounts by the body, but one that has an incredibly important job. Its one key role is it helps insulin work more efficiently. This seemingly minor role has tremendous effects for preserving and improving health throughout the body. Unfortunately, most people don't get the tiny amounts of chromium they need from their diets.

As you've learned, supplementing the diet with chromium can offer widespread health benefits. Chromium protects against a long laundry list of common health problems, including two top killers in our society—diabetes and cardiovascular disease. Chromium slows down aging. It normalizes blood sugar function and staves off carbohydrate cravings. It regulates blood cholesterol profiles, lowering the bad types and increasing the good. It combats Syndrome X and helps improve body composition. It alleviates some types of depression and premenstrual syndrome. And it improves bone health and helps prevent osteoporosis.

Although chromium sounds like a panacea and too good to be true, it isn't. Chromium offers all these benefits because it helps insulin works more efficiently. Insulin that works efficiently does the rest.

The most common health maladies facing our society today are disorders of inefficient blood sugar and insulin function. Any nutrient that improves blood sugar and insulin function turns out to be an all-star nutrient. That's exactly what chromium is.

It's time now to weigh the evidence and use this information to your advantage. Make the decision to fortify yourself with supplemental chromium and let this mighty mineral work for you.

SELECTED
REFERENCES

Anderson, RA. Chromium, glucose intolerance and diabetes. *Journal of the American College of Nutrition,* 1998; 17:548–555.

Anderson, RA, Bryden, NA, Polansky, MM. Dietary chromium intake. Freely chosen diets, institutional diet, and individual foods. *Biological Trace Element Research,* 1992; 32:117–121.

Anderson, RA, Bryden, NA, Polansky, MM. Lack of toxicity of chromium chloride and chromium picolinate in rats. *Journal of the American College of Nutrition,* 1997; 16:273–279.

Anderson, RA, Chen, N, Bryden, NA, et al. Elevated intakes of supplemental chromium improve glucose and insulin variables in individuals with type 2 diabetes. *Diabetes,* 1997; 46:1786–1791.

Anderson, RA, Kozlovsky, AS. Chromium intake, absorption and excretion of subjects consuming self-selected diets. *American Journal of Clinical Nutrition,* 1985; 41:1177–1183.

Anderson, RA, Polasky, MM, Bryden, NA, et al. Effects of supplemental chromium on patients with symptoms of reactive hypoglycemia. *Metabolism,* 1987; 36:351–355.

Cefalu, WT, Bell-Farrow, AD, Stegner, J, et al. Effect of chromium picolinate on insulin sensitivity in vivo. *The Journal of Trace Elements in Experimental Medicine,* 1999; 12:71–83.

Cheng, N, Zhu, X, Shi, H, et al. Follow-up survey of people in China with type 2 diabetes mellitus consuming supplemental chromium. *The Journal of Trace Elements in Experimental Medicine,* 1999; 12:55–60.

Evans, GW, Meyer, LK. Life span is increased in rats supplemented with a chromium-pyridine 2 carboxylate complex. *Advances in Scientific Research,* 1994; 1:19–23.

Evans, GW, Swenson, G, Walters, K. Chromium picolinate decreases calcium excretion and increases dehydroepiandrosterone (DHEA) in post menopausal women. *FASEB Journal,* 1995; 9:525.

Jovanovic-Petersen, L, Gutierrez, M, Peterson, CM. Chromium supplementation for gestational diabetic women improves glucose tolerance and decreases hyperinsulinemia. *Journal of the American College of Nutrition,* 1995; 14:530.

Kaats, GR, Blum, K, Pullin, D, et al. A randomized, double-masked, placebo-controlled study of the effects of chromium picolinate supplementation of body composition: a replication and extension of a previous study. *Current Therapeutic Research,* 1998; 59:379–388.

Kaats, GR, Keith, SC, Wise, JA, et al. Effects of baseline total cholesterol levels on diet and exercise interventions. *Journal of the American Nutraceutical Association,* 1999; 2:42–49.

Khan, A, Bryden, NA, Polansky, MM, et al. Insulin potentiating factor and chromium content of selected foods and spices. *Biological Trace Element Research,* 1990; 24:183–188.

Komoroski, J, Greenberg, D, Maki, KC, et al. Chromium picolinate with biotin attenuates elevation in blood glucose levels in people with type 2 diabetes ingesting medium carbohydrate nutritional beverages. Presented at the 2001 American College of Nutrition Annual Meeting, October 6, 2001, Orlando, Florida.

Lane, BC. Myopia prevention and reversal: new data confirms the interaction of accommodative stress and deficit-inducing nutrition. *Journal of the International Academy of Preventive Medicine*, 1982; VII:17–30.

Lee, NA, and Reasner, CA. Beneficial effect of chromium supplementation on serum triglyceride levels in NIDDM. *Diabetes Care*, 1994; 17:1449–1452.

McCarthy, M. High-chromium yeast for acne? *Medical Hypothesis*, 1984; 14:307–310.

McLeod, MN, Gaynes, BN, Golden, RN. Chromium potentiation of antidepressant pharmacotherapy for dysthymic disorder in 5 patients. *Journal of Clinical Psychiatry*, 1999; 60:237–240.

McLeod, MN, Golden, RN. Chromium treatment of depression. *International Journal of Neuropsychopharmacology*, 2000; 3:311–314.

Preuss, HG, Jarrell, ST, Scheckenbach, R, et al. Comparative effects of chromium, vanadium and gymnema sylvestre on sugar-induced blood pressure elevations in SHR. *Journal of the American College of Nutrition*, 1998; 17:116–123.

Ravina, A, Slezak, L, Mirsky, N, et al. Reversal of corticosteroid-induced diabetes mellitus with supplemental chromium. *Diabetic Medicine*, 1999; 16:164–167.

Ravina, A, Slezak, L, Rubal, A, et al. Clinical use of the trace element chromium (III) in the treatment of diabetes mellitus. *The Journal of Trace Elements in Experimental Medicine*, 1995; 8:183–190.

OTHER BOOKS AND RESOURCES

Broadhurst, C. Leigh. *Diabetes: Prevention and Cure*. New York, NY: Kensington Books, 1999.
An easy-to-read book that offers a wealth of information for those with type II or type I diabetes. It outlines a diet and supplement approach to their treatment, which includes chromium supplements.

Challem, Jack, Berkson, Burton, and Smith, Melissa Diane. *Syndrome X: The Complete Nutritional Program to Prevent and Reverse Insulin Resistance*. New York, NY: John Wiley & Sons, 2000.
The definitive consumer guide to Syndrome X—the combination of insulin resistance with abdominal obesity, high cholesterol, high triglycerides, and high blood pressure—which sets the stage for heart disease, type II diabetes, and other degenerative diseases. The book includes therapeutic diets, recipes, and supplement plans involving chromium for this common condition.

Challem, Jack, and Brown, Liz. *User's Guide to Vitamins and Minerals*. North Bergen, NJ: Basic Health Books, 2002.
A reader-friendly guide that covers the basics of all vit-amins and minerals that are essential for health, from A to zinc.

Challem, Jack, and Smith, Melissa Diane. *User's Guide to Vitamin E*. North Bergen, NJ: Basic Health Books, 2002.
A reader-friendly guide that covers the basics of heart-protective vitamin E.

Smith, Melissa Diane. *Going Against the Grain: How Reducing and Avoiding Grains Can Revitalize Your Health.* Chicago, Illinois: Contemporary Books, 2002.

A book that covers all the health problems that can result from eating too many grains (and sugars), including conditions such as Syndrome X, overweight, and diabetes, as well as gluten sensitivity, grain allergies, and autoimmune disorders. Three therapeutic diets are outlined, along with information on supplements (including chromium) that are helpful for various conditions.

GreatLife Magazine
Consumer magazine with articles on vitamins, minerals, herbs, and foods.

Available for free at many health and natural food stores.

Let's Live Magazine
Consumer magazine with emphasis on the health benefits of vitamins, minerals, and herbs.

Customer service:
1-800-676-4333
P.O. Box 74908
Los Angeles, CA 90004

Subscriptions: 12 issues per year, $19.95 in the U.S.; $31.95 outside the U.S.

Physical Magazine
Magazine oriented to body builders and other serious athletes.

Customer service:
1-800-676-4333
P.O. Box 74908
Los Angeles, CA 90004

Subscriptions: 12 issues per year, $19.95 in the U.S.; $31.95 outside the U.S.

The Nutrition Reporter™ newsletter

Monthly newsletter that summarizes recent medical research on vitamins, minerals, and herbs.

Customer service:

P.O. Box 30246

Tucson, AZ 85751-0246

e-mail: jack@thenutritionreporter.com

www.nutritionreporter.com

Subscriptions: $26 per year (12 issues) in the U.S.; $32 U.S. or $48 CNC for Canada; $38 for other countries

The Chromium Information Bureau Website

A not-for-profit educational organization that provides information to consumers, health care providers, nutrition researchers, and the media about the clinical functions, effects, and actions of dietary chromium.

P.O. Box 107

Inglefield, IN 47618

www.chromiuminfo.org

Index

Acne, 52–53

Adult-onset diabetes. *See* Diabetes, type II.

Advanced glycation end-products. *See* AGEs.

AGEs, 29, 33

Aging, 1, 7, 27–34, 78

Alcoholism, 48–49

Alpha-lipoic acid, 71–72

Alzheimer's disease, 51

Anderson, Richard, 19

Antidepressant drugs, 36, 41

 selective serotonin reuptake inhibitors, 36–37, 42, 49

 tricyclic, 36

Atypical features (Depression), 41

Biotin, 73

Blood pressure, 17, 20–21

Blood sugar, 3, 4, 5, 6, 7, 10–16, 27–34, 35, 40, 45, 52, 57, 58, 73, 76, 80

Bulimia, 48–50

Caloric intake, 30–31

Cancer, 4, 51

Carbohydrates, 18–22, 23–26, 50, 53, 67, 76–77

Carnitine, 75

Cataracts, 29

Cefalu, William, 14

Chelator, 59

Chicago Center for Clinical Research, 74

Cholesterol, 17–22, 73. *See also* HDL; LDL.

Chromium, 1–87

 and other nutrients, 68–79

 chelated, 59

 choosing, 61–67

 definition, 3

 doctors opinions, 64–65

 dosages, 7, 8, 13, 14, 38, 63–64

 excretion of, 8

 foods and, 8

 industrial, 4

 nutritional, 3, 4,

 research, 30, 37–39, 46–47

 safety, 60

 scientific support for, 64

 shopping for, 57–67

side effects, 61
Chromium picolinate, 12, 13, 19, 21, 25, 38, 47, 59, 60, 74
CLA. *See* Conjugated linoleic acid.
Colorado State University, 51
Conjugated linoleic acid, 72
Cordain, Loren, 51
Corticosteroids, 15
Cortisol, 20

Dehydroepiandrosterone. *See* DHEA.
Depression, 1, 35–45. *See also* Atypical features.
DHEA, 31–32, 46–47, 78
Diabetes, 1, 2, 5, 10–16, 17–22, 27–34, 80
  gestational, 15
  type I, 10, 14
  type II, 10–16, 27–34, 47, 55, 57, 63, 74, 77
Diabetes mellitus, 11
Diachrome, 73
Diet, 76
Duke University, 39
Dysthymia, 35–36

Endocrine glands, 32
Estrogen, 48
Erin Brokovich, 4
Exercise, 78
Evans, Gary, 46–47, 59
Eyesight, 53–54

FASEB Journal, 46

Fat, 77–78
Fat metabolism, 18–19
Fatty acids, 71
FDA. *See* Food and Drug Administration.
Food and Drug Administration, 5
Food and Nutrition Board of the National Research Council, 5
Free radicals, 28, 33

Garcinia cambogia, 75
Glucagon, 77
Glucose. *See* Blood sugar.
Glucose tolerance factor, 58
Glycosylated hemoglobin. *See* Hemoglobin A1c.
GTF. *See* Glucose tolerance factor.

HCA. *See* Hydroxycitric acid.
HDL, 7, 17–22
Headaches, 61
Heart disease, 17, 27, 80
Hemoglobin A1c, 12, 16, 29
Hepatothermic effect, 75
Hereditary hemachroma - tosis. *See* Iron overload.
Hexavalent chromium. *See* Chromium, industrial.
Hormones, 32–33, 54
Hydroxycitric acid, 75
Hypertension, 20, 37
Hypoglycemia, 15, 63
  reactive, 15–16

Infertility, 54–55
Insulin, 1, 2, 5, 6, 7, 10–16,
    17–22, 23–26, 27–34,
    40, 45, 46–47, 51, 52,
    54–55, 76–77, 80
Insulin resistance, 6–7, 14,
    18–21, 23–26, 46–47,
    51, 54–55, 70
Iron overload, 56, 71

Joints, 29
*Journal of Clinical
    Psychiatry*, 38
*Journal of the International
    Academy of Preventive
    Medicine*, 53
Juvenile-onset diabetes.
    See Diabetes, type I.

Kaats, Gilbert, 19

Lane, Benjamin, 53–54
LDL, 17, 18
Lean body mass, 24–25

Magnesium, 70
MAOIs, 36, 41
McLeod, Malcolm, 37–44,
    49, 61
Metabolic makeover, 75
Minerals, 3, 65, 70–71
    definition, 3
    nutritional, 3
    trace, 3
    See also Supplements.
Molecular docks, 6
Monoamine oxidase
    inhibitors. *See* MAOIs.
Multivitamins, 65–66

Nearsightedness, 53–54
Neurotransmitters, 40
*New England Journal of
    Medicine*, 32
Niacin. *See* Vitamin B_3.
Norepinephrine, 40
Nutrients, 68–79

Obesity, 2, 17, 21–22,
    23–26, 75
    upper body, 17, 21
Omega-3, 71
Osteoporosis, 1, 46–48
Ovarian cysts, 54–55
Overweight, 2, 17, 21–22,
    23–26

PCOS. *See* Polycystic
    ovary syndrome.
PMS. *See* Premenstrual
    syndrome.
Polycystic ovary
    syndrome, 54–55
Postmenopause, 31, 36,
    46–48
Postnatal depression, 36
Pregnancy, 15
Premenstrual syndrome,
    1, 36, 38, 41–42, 44
    research, 42
Protein, 77
Prozac, 36

QVC home shopping
    channel, 75

Recommended Daily
    Allowance
    Committee, 7

SAD. *See* Seasonal
    affective disorder.
Seasonal affective
    disorder, 1, 36, 42–43
Serotonin, 40, 43–44
Silymarin, 71–72
Skin, 29, 52–53
Skin diabetes, 52
Sleep, 78
Sleep apnea, 55
Sodium, 20
Spices, 78
SSRI antidepressants. *See*
    Antidepressant drugs.
St. John's wort, 44
Stress reduction, 78–79
Sugar levels, 27–26
Suicide, 36
Supplements, 9, 14, 22,
    34, 57–67
  child use, 63
  choosing, 61
  dosages, 13, 58, 63
  form, 58–59
  purchasing, 57–67
  results gauging, 21, 22
Syndrome X, 17–22, 47,
    49, 55, 56, 57, 63, 69,
    74, 80. *See also*
    Glucose.
*Syndrome X: The
    Complete Nutritional
    Program to Prevent
    and Reverse Insulin
    Resistance*, 22

Thiazide diuretics, 15
TPN. *See* Total Parental
    Nutrition.
Total Parental Nutrition, 4
Triglycerides, 7, 17
Trivalent chromium. *See*
    Chromium, nutritional.
Tryptophan, 40

University of North
    Carolina, Chapel Hill,
    37–40
University of Vermont
    College of Medicine,
    73–74
University of Wisconsin,
    Madison, 30

Violence, 36
Vitamin B complex,
    69–70
Vitamin B_3, 73
Vitamin C, 68–69
Vitamin E, 68–69
Vitamins, 3, 65. *See also*
    Supplements.

Weight control, 24–25
Winter blues, 42–43

Yeast, high-chromium,
    52–53

Zinc, 70
Zoloft, 36

Printed in the USA
CPSIA information can be obtained
at www.ICGtesting.com
JSHW012008140824
68134JS00004B/79

9 781681 628462